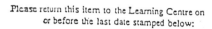

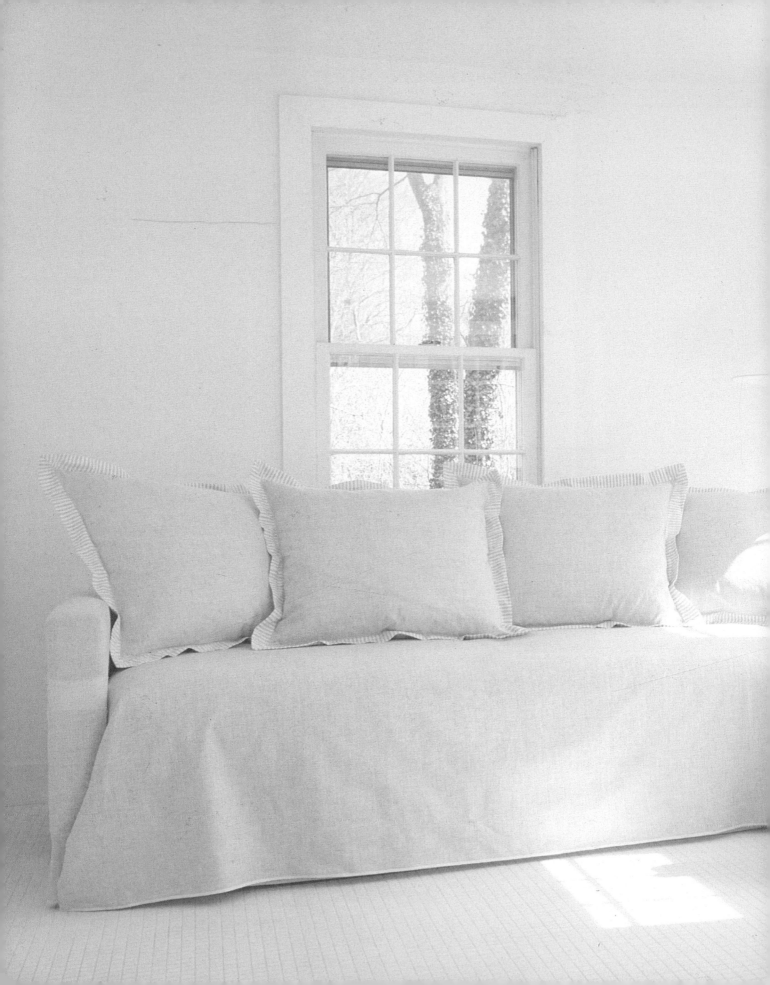

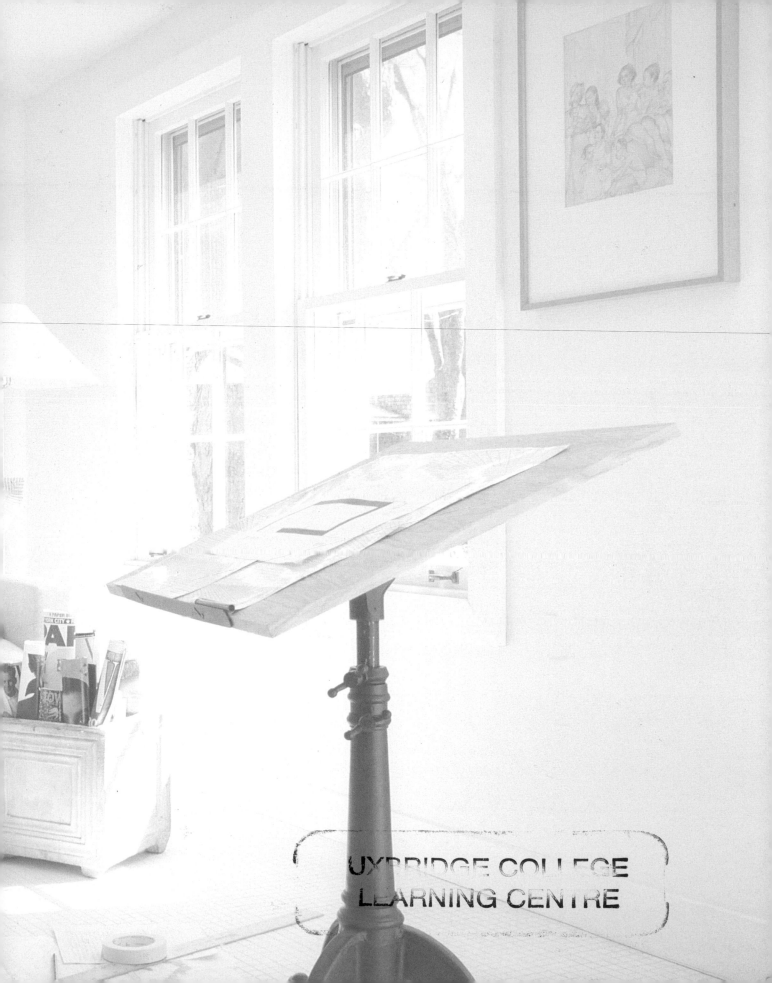

the
allergy-free
home

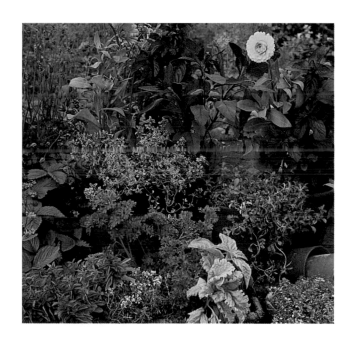

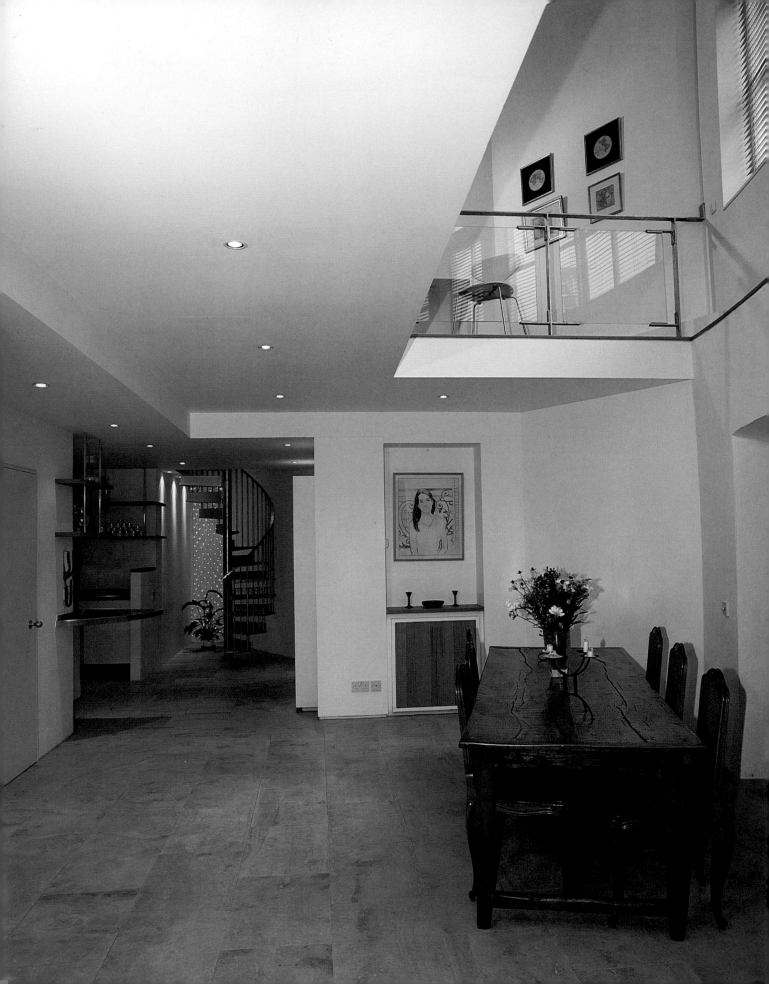

the allergy-free home

A practical guide to creating a healthy environment

VITTORIA D'ALESSIO

APPLE

Printed and bound in Singapore

Volume copyright © 2001 Breslich & Foss Ltd

Text copyright © 2001 by Vittoria D'Alessio

Illustration copyright © 2001 by Trina Dalziel

ISBN 1-84092-346-6

A catalogue record for this book is available from the British Library.

APPLE

First published in the United Kingdom by
Apple Press
Sheridan House
4th Floor
112-116A Western Road
Hove
E. Sussex BN3 1DD

This book was conceived and produced by
Breslich & Foss Ltd
20 Wells Mews
London W1T 3HQ

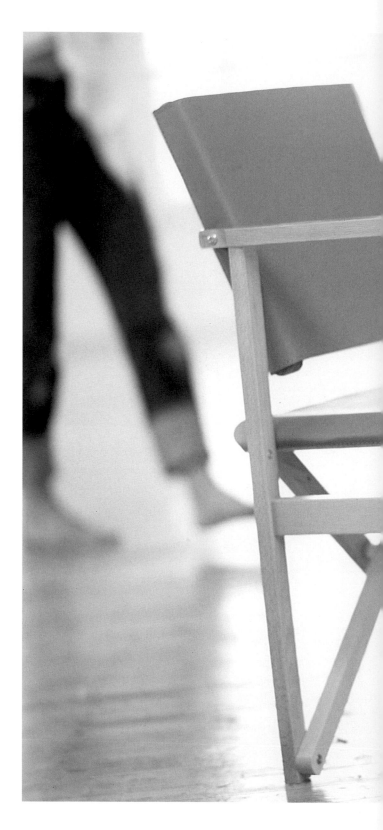

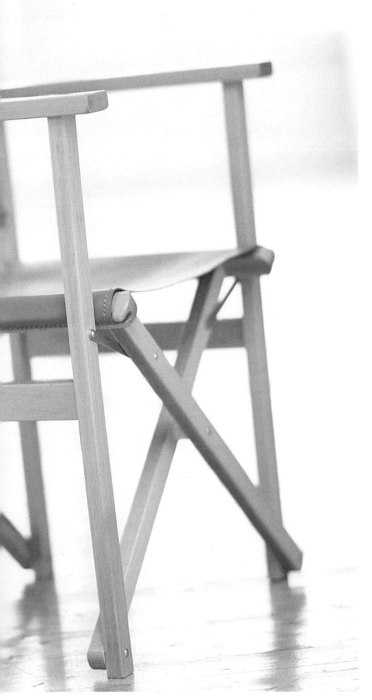

contents

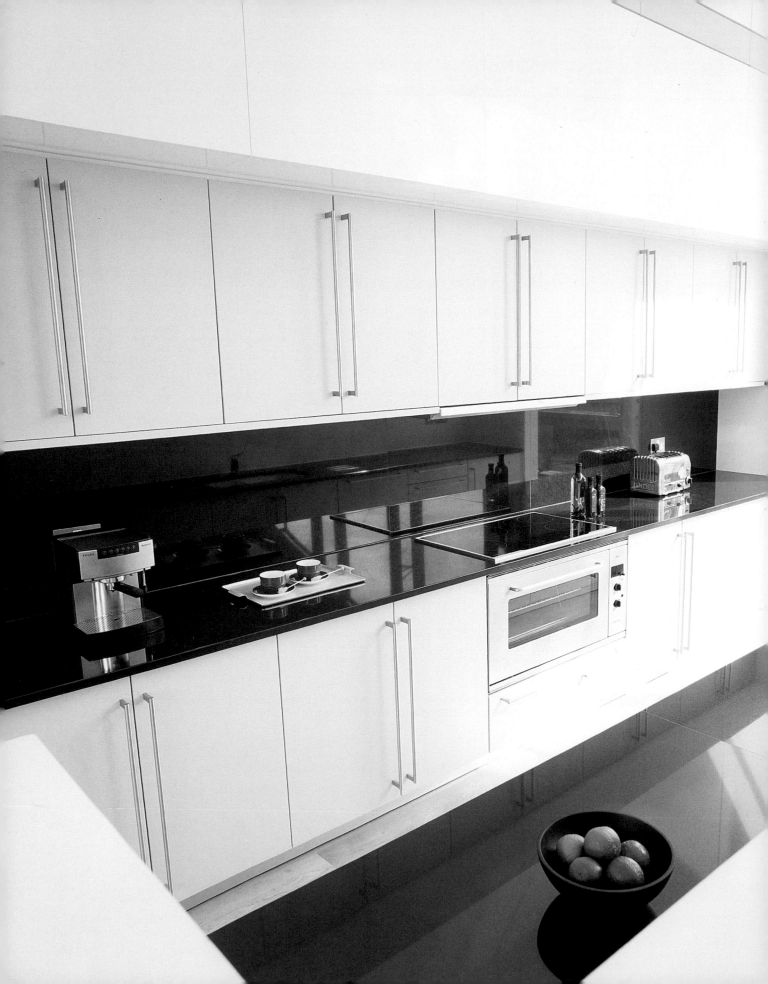

Foreword

The industrialised world is facing an allergy epidemic. For the past 40 years, there has been a startling increase in both humdrum and exotic auto-immune responses to our environment, and it is now estimated that one in three people suffers from some form of allergy. Whatever the root cause of the allergy plague, the fact that indoor pollution is a major – perhaps even the main – contributing factor is fast gaining acceptance among allergy experts.

The focus of this book is on the positive steps that each one of us can take to reduce allergy-causing problems within the home with a minimum of expense and disruption. For example, advice is given on the many simple changes you can make to your household environment that will dramatically reduce the indoor air pollutants believed to trigger allergic disorders; there is precise cleaning information regarding dust mites and moulds; and a list of non-allergenic indoor plants. You will also find recipes for safe and natural cleaning products.

What I hope to achieve in *The Allergy-Free Home* is to demonstrate that the battle against indoor allergens is worth fighting, and that it can be fought one manageable step at a time.

Vittoria D'Alessio

Introduction

Fifty years ago, it was unusual to meet someone with an allergy. Today between a quarter and a half of the population of developed countries are affected. It is not fully understood why some people develop allergies and others don't: DNA can't explain the rise, merely why one person is more likely than another to develop an allergy. There is clearly something else going on that is responsible for this trend.

On closer examination it becomes clear that the explosion of allergies coincides with the economic miracle of the 1950s and 60s, and that allergic disease is a growing problem only in first-world countries. The United Kingdom has the highest prevalence of asthma symptoms in 13 to 14 year olds in the world, followed by Australia, New Zealand, the Republic of Ireland and the USA. The lowest prevalence, according to the survey's findings, is in Eastern European countries, North Africa and India. To many people, this sort of statistic will come as a surprise: allergy – and asthma in particular – is widely regarded as an urban phenomenon linked to car fumes and industry, so it seems odd that it should be rife in Australia and New Zealand, where green space is plentiful and outdoor pollution relatively low. The idea that outdoor pollution is **not** a major factor in the development of allergic disease is gaining acceptance. Instead, events that occur indoors, in the home in particular, appear to be largely to blame. Given that most of us spend an estimated 90 per cent of every day indoors and just 5 per cent outside (the rest is spent in transit), we are all at considerable risk.

THE MODERN, AIRTIGHT HOME

Without a doubt, our predilection for cosy, densely furnished rooms is largely to blame for the upward spiral of allergic disease. Warm, centrally heated rooms, wall-to-wall carpets, thick curtains, upholstered sofas, fluffy cushions and premium bedding material all provide deluxe living conditions for the pesky and highly allergy-forming

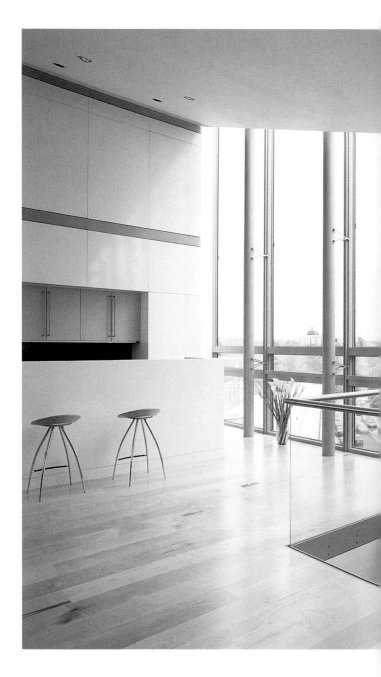

house-dust mite. Pets are another allergy time-bomb, yet few contemporary buildings provide adequate ventilation to dispel the allergy-forming particles that are shed by resident furry mammals. A third common source of allergic disease is mould, which is prevalent in the modern home for the simple reason that newer buildings are more airtight. Condensation builds up faster, and mould gets the perfect damp environment in which to flourish.

THE SYNTHETIC HOME

Dust mites, pets and mould are easily the most recognisable allergy triggers in the home, but they are by no means the only ones. There is substantial evidence – particularly from Scandinavian countries – that a vast array of synthetic products used indoors are also contributing to the rise in allergies and allergy-like disorders. These products include household chemicals, synthetic fabrics, DIY products, cosmetics, pesticides, tobacco smoke, over-the-counter medicines and emissions from gas cooking. Some are absorbed through the skin; others enter our bodies when we breathe then pass into the lungs, where they either remain or are absorbed into the bloodstream.

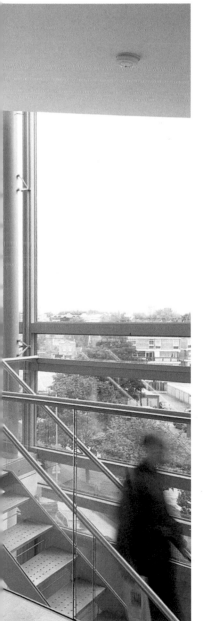

At present, research projects looking at the health implications of indoor air pollution are funded at around one tenth of the level of those concerned with outdoor pollution. As a direct consequence of this under-funding, we now find ourselves in a situation where many people are exposed to man-made substances in the home that would not be tolerated at work or outdoors.

THE HYGIENE HYPOTHESIS

According to proponents of the so-called 'Hygiene Hypothesis', we live in a world that is obsessed with cleanliness. Our bodies encounter

LEFT A home free of clutter, curtains, and carpets provides the perfect backdrop for an allergy-free lifestyle.

BELOW Allergy sufferers should keep man-made fabrics, such as nylon and MDF, to a minimum, opting for natural fabrics and wood instead – though allergen barrier covers should be used on some natural materials.

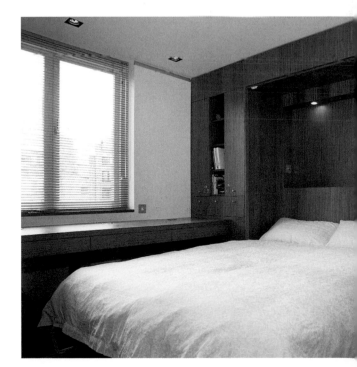
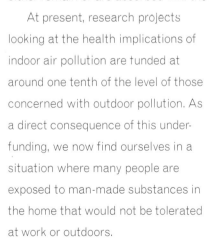

fewer microbes in daily life and our immune systems have started to tilt away from a protective response towards an allergic one. In other words, the very measures taken to enhance health have backfired, making us less able to stave off allergies. Lending weight to this theory is the fact that younger siblings who are more exposed to infection are less likely to develop allergies than only children.

According to the small print of this popular hypothesis, modern hygiene comes in various guises: we live in over-sanitised premises; we avoid disease through vaccinations; we extinguish bacterial infections with antibiotics before our immune systems have mounted a satisfactory response; we eat food that is highly sterile.

Overly sterile food is thought to be harmful because it lacks the microbes that in times past promoted the proliferation of gut flora, the so-called 'friendly' bacteria that stimulated the immune system in a way that lent protection against allergies. Scientists believe we may soon be giving babies 'live' inoculations that will expose them to bacteria they do not encounter in the hygienic home.

THE EXOTIC DIET

Doctors are mystified by the explosion of food allergies in developed societies. The most convincing theory to date is that our guts are simply poorly adapted to cope with the variety of exotic ingredients found in the modern diet. If the theory holds true, though we have become culturally familiar with exotic foods, our bodies have failed to keep apace, and food allergies surface when our immune systems regard a new ingredient as 'alien' and therefore an 'enemy'.

THE MISSING LINK

All the risk factors discussed above have been implicated in the onset of allergic disease and the flare-up of pre-existing conditions, but no one knows the full story and no single factor stands out as the overriding cause of allergy. The likelihood of a person developing an allergic condition is almost certainly determined by a series of interrelated

factors, and even specialists are left guessing what all of these might be. The problem may be complicated by, say, the number of baths we take in a week, the frequency with which we wash our clothes or the way we keep fit. These, however, are merely stabs in the dark.

But why worry about the undiscovered segments of the puzzle when there are so many known and heavily suspected risk factors? Allergy cannot be cured, but in many cases it can be prevented. And by focusing on prevention – identifying and reducing allergy triggers – it is often possible to stop allergic disease from developing in the first place (primary prevention) and to ease the symptoms of pre-existing allergies (secondary prevention).

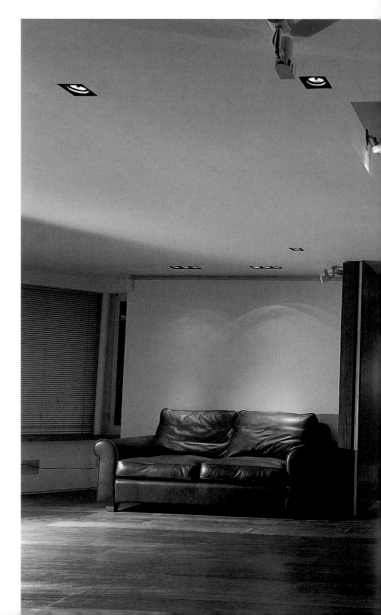

HOW TO USE THIS BOOK

Many people suspect they have an allergy but cannot give it a name. Others know what to call their condition but can't list the substances that trigger their symptoms. The chances are that many allergy sufferers don't know how to avoid triggers without turning their homes into hospital wards. This book aims to guide affected individuals through the stages of naming and understanding allergies, with the ultimate aim of providing a framework for change, leading to a more satisfactory quality of life.

The list of 'symptoms' displayed in the opening section of chapter 1 guides people in the early stages of allergy awareness towards a likely diagnosis (though it must be stressed that conventional medical tests should always be sought to confirm or refute self-diagnosis). Next comes a full discussion on allergies – what they are and how they are thought to arise – followed by an explanation of the latest medical tests on offer to help people identify the specific particles or substances in their environment or diet that trigger allergic reactions. Chapter 2 examines the known and suspected 'causes' or 'triggers' of allergies and allergy-like conditions. And in the final chapter, there are dozens of suggestions that can be applied in the home to reduce the symptoms of allergy and allergy-like conditions, and in some cases to eliminate them (though not neces sarily the underlying allergy) altogether.

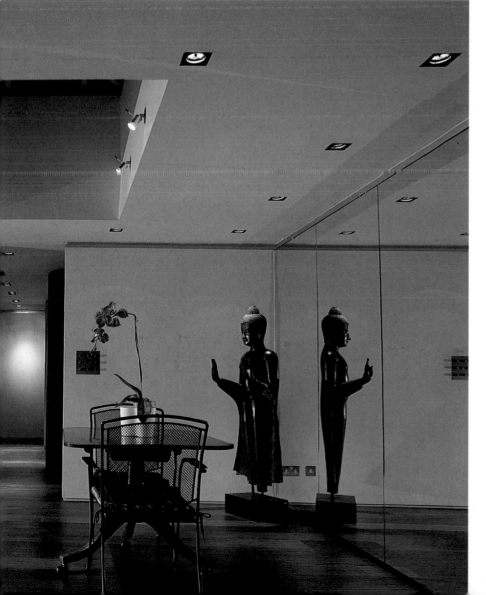

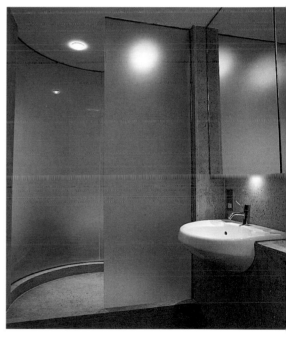

ABOVE Keep the decor simple and natural in the bathroom. Favour easy-to-clean materials such as tiles, glass, wood and ceramic.

LEFT Leather chairs and sofas make an excellent (though costly) alternative to upholstered soft furnishings for allergy sufferers. Dust mites can be simply wiped off. And if you aspire to a natural lifestyle, you can't beat real hide.

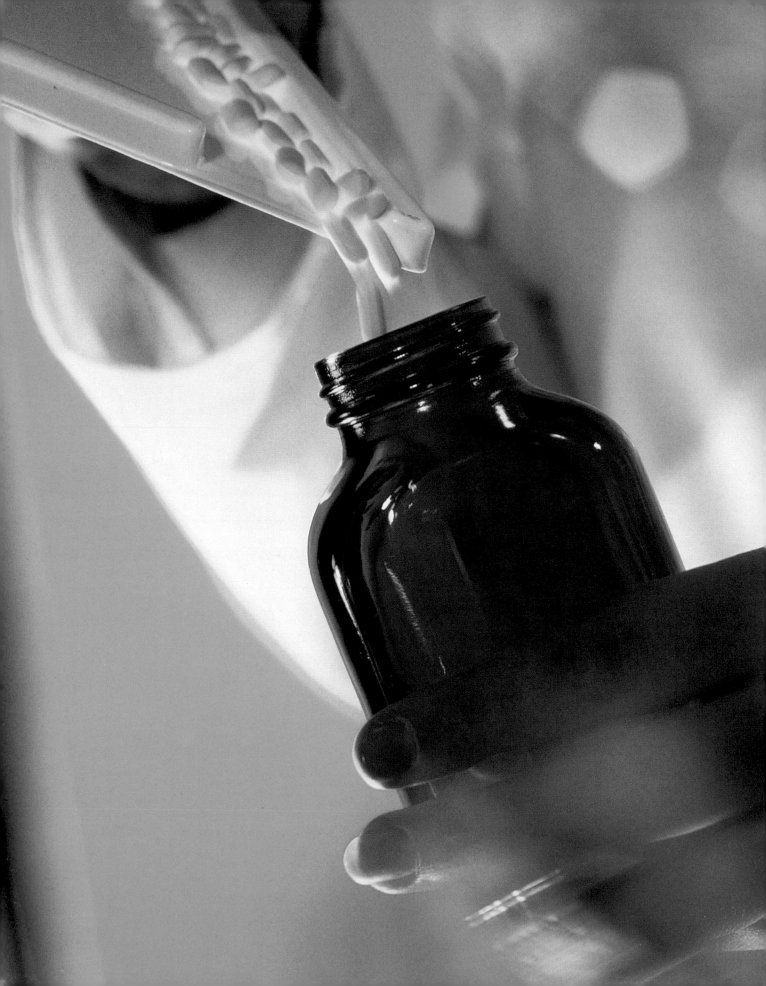

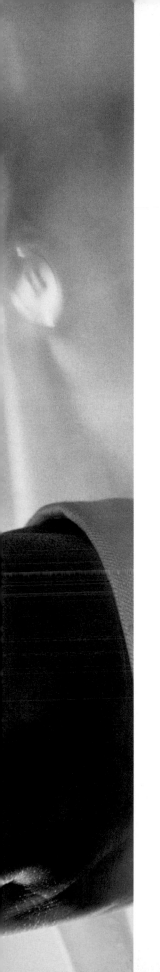

symptoms, diagnosis and treatment

An allergic reaction occurs when the body's immune system overreacts to a normally harmless substance; for example, a protein in a food or a drug. This reaction causes symptoms that range from a runny nose and itchy eyes to laboured breathing and a skin rash. An allergy can cause extreme irritation and disability, aggravating the senses of smell, sight, taste and touch. At worst, it can be fatal.

The immune system responds to the substance perceived as harmful by producing a specific antibody to fight it. This antibody is called Immunoglobulin E, or IgE. The next time the body encounters the offending substance, the immune system 'remembers' it from the previous exposure and produces more IgE. This attaches itself to cells in our bodies, the most important of which are mast cells, which then burst and release histamine, cytokines, leukotrienes and other chemicals into the bloodstream. These released substances are what cause the irritation, inflammation and many other symptoms of an allergic response.

WHAT IS AN ALLERGEN?

The substances in the environment that cause allergic reactions are known as allergens. Almost anything can be an allergen for someone, though easily the most common allergens are house-dust mites, pollen, pets, stinging insects and some foods. It is actually protein in the offending substance that causes an allergic reaction. There are, however, some allergens – such as penicillin – that contain no protein; these substances must become bound to a protein inside the body in order to elicit an immune response.

It is not just the initial introduction of an allergen into a person's life that determines whether or not an allergy will develop. Other contributing factors are: the concentration of the allergen; repeated exposure to the allergen; exposure to multiple allergens; the pre-existence of other non-airborne allergies; and the use of some medicines. Exposure to allergens at certain vulnerable times, such as during pregnancy or after a viral infection, seems to contribute to the development of allergies.

ALLERGY TRIGGERS

'Trigger' is the term used for any substance or situation that sparks the symptoms of an allergy. Every person with an allergy or intolerance is sensitive to different triggers, and learning to avoid the relevant ones is an important step in managing the existing condition. A trigger may be an allergen or some other irritant. Common triggers include colds, flu and other viral infections; exercise, cold air, cigarette smoke, foods, certain do-it-yourself materials, house-hold chemicals and perfumes. There are many others.

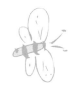

MULTIPLE CHEMICAL SENSITIVITY

This condition is sometimes known as 'allergy to life' and describes a person who has become ultrasensitive to chemicals either through a single high-level exposure or through continuous low-level exposure in the home. Once damage is done to the immune system, exposure to all sorts of chemicals can trigger symptoms. Around 15 per cent of people in the UK and 17 per cent of people in Australia are believed to suffer from increased sensitivity to chemicals.

INTOLERANCES AND SENSITIVITIES

Some people have exaggerated, allergy-like reactions to substances they routinely encounter in their lives. These substances may be natural or synthetic and include perfumes, cosmetics, fresh paint, new carpeting, household chemicals and pesticides. Though the symptoms resemble those associated with allergies, chemical sensitivities do not involve IgE or histamine, and are therefore not classed as true allergic responses.

It is seldom helpful to tell a person with a sensitivity that his or her symptoms do not amount to an allergy; the implication is that the condition is trivial. As there is considerable overlap between allergy triggers and sensitivity triggers, this book covers both types of reaction. However, allergies and sensitivities are managed and treated very differently, so at the time of diagnosis it is essential to view the two as distinct.

SENSITISATION

This term describes the process by which a body's immune system comes to recognise and then react to something in the environment. Sensitisation occurs after an introductory exposure to the offending substance or particle. Subsequent encounters with the offending matter result in the body mounting an allergic or allergy-like response.

FAMILY HISTORY

There are two important risk factors for developing allergies: the environment (e.g. allergens in a person's home) and genetic make-up. If one parent suffers from allergies, there is a 30 to 50 per cent chance he or she will pass that tendency on to his or her child (the link is strongest between mothers and babies). If both parents suffer from allergies, the probability rises to 60 to 80 per cent. Within a family, allergies often co-exist, so if a close relative has an allergy, you are more likely to develop another. This is because parents pass on an overall tendency to develop allergies, not a specific sensitivity to a given allergen. The tendency is probably to produce lots of IgE. The inherited likelihood to develop allergies can result in the emergence of symptoms later in life, not just in childhood.

The word 'atopic' describes a group of allergic diseases that often affect several members of a family. Allergies that typically display this hereditary trait include atopic dermatitis, allergic rhinitis and asthma. However, 20 per cent of people with atopic allergic conditions are the only ones in their families to be affected.

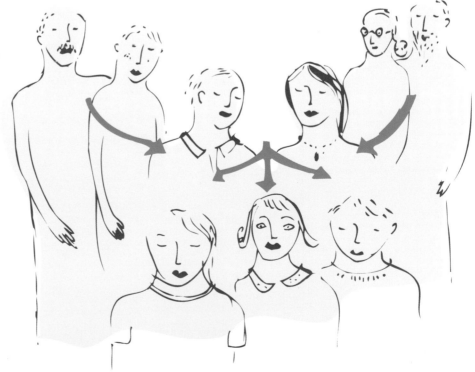

CHILDREN

From birth, a baby who goes
on to develop allergies shows
a different immune response
from other newborns, which
leads allergy experts to
believe something
happens during pregnancy
to direct a foetus down the
allergic pathway. Research
at Southampton University
is concentrating on a mother's
immune response during
pregnancy, and it is possible that in
generations to come, pregnant women
will be advised to restrict their exposure to
common allergens.

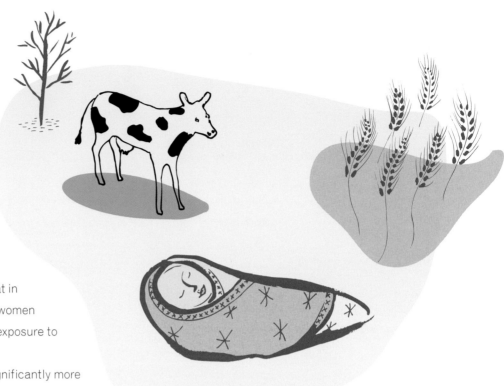

Predisposed children are significantly more
likely to develop allergies if they are exposed to
high levels of allergens in infancy, when their
immune systems are undergoing critical stages of development. Until recently it was believed that babies who
were exclusively breastfed during their first four months of
life gained some protection from allergies; however, new
research suggests this is only true for atopic eczema, and
then only if the lactating mother avoids foods linked with
childhood eczema, such as cow's milk and eggs.

FOOD ALLERGY IN INFANTS

Although almost any food is a potential
allergen, the following foods are most
likely to trigger a reaction in infants:
egg white, cow's milk protein, wheat,
peanuts, sesame, bony fish, citrus fruits
and soy protein.

ALLERGIES IN THE ELDERLY

Doctors tend to see fewer allergies among the elderly. This
is probably because anyone born between 50 and 70 years
ago was less likely to encounter allergy triggers in their
early days and was therefore less likely to develop an
allergy as an adult.

Often, people who are diagnosed with an allergy later
in life remember having breathing problems, or even
asthma, as children. In other cases, childhood allergies
remain a presence throughout a person's life, though
symptoms tend to become less intense in old age.
New allergies can, nonetheless, emerge at any age, and
'late-onset' allergy is becoming more common. In older
people, it can be difficult for a doctor to make a diagnosis
of asthma, as the symptoms can be similar to other lung
diseases or even to heart disease. Sometimes asthma co-
exists with one or more of these conditions.

SESAME

Sesame allergy affects about one in two thousand people in the United Kingdom, and after peanuts is the second most severe food allergy. In Australia, where sesame was only recently introduced as a common food, the number of children with an allergy to it is greater than it is for nuts.

Foods that contain sesame include hummus, tahini, halva, some breads and many Greek and Mexican products. It is also sold as a cooking and seasoning oil. It is even used in cosmetics (as *Sesamum Indicum L*). Severely allergic individuals should avoid sesame in all forms.

FOOD ALLERGY AND INTOLERANCE

Many people experience negative reactions to certain ingredients in their diets, but only 20 per cent actually have a truly demonstrable allergic reaction. In the remainder, the reaction is in fact a manifestation of a food intolerance. Symptoms usually clear up when the offending foods are removed from the diet.

For a food allergy to develop, the allergen must penetrate the gut wall, triggering an immune response to the foreign food protein. This is followed by sensitisation to that protein. In healthy individuals, the body successfully protects itself against allergen penetration by two important means: an antibody found in the gut called secretory IgA reduces gut penetration of food allergens, and gut enzymes (whose job it is to degrade food) reduce the potency of allergens. People with a food allergy often have one of two faults in their protective mechanisms: either an IgA deficiency or an inflammatory disease that weakens intestinal barriers. Reactions can occur to tiny traces of the offending food, which is most allergenic in the fresh form. Cooking reduces or eliminates its potency.

Food allergies are most likely to occur in infancy because babies have an immature gut, which means they digest less efficiently and they are more likely to have a breach in the integrity of their bowels. As the gastrointestinal surface barrier naturally improves with age, the incidence of food allergy tends to decrease and is usually resolved by the age of three.

In adults, the most common allergens are bony fish, shellfish, peanuts, tree-nuts, tomatoes and chocolate. Less common allergens include strawberries, oranges, peaches, coconut, beef, pork, sesame, nuts (hazel, cashew, almonds, Brazil), beans, mustard, celery, potatoes and peas.

FOOD LABELS

Studies suggest that 0.5 per cent of children in Australia and 2 per cent of children in the UK have a peanut allergy, and symptoms are frequently severe. Such is the public fear of nut allergies that many companies now print a disclaimer on their products stating 'This product may contain nut traces', even if the presence of a nut particle is very unlikely. This precaution has arisen from the fact that a severe allergic reaction may be triggered by the tiniest trace of nut, and even when production lines are kept scrupulously clean, the risk of contamination remains. The result is that an ever-decreasing selection of foods is certified as safe. However, a small number of companies offer products that are guaranteed nut-free.

Do bear in mind that sometimes a processed food product may undergo a tweaking to its formula, which means that previously safe food may become dangerous to allergy sufferers. Never assume a food is safe to eat just because you have had it before; always check the label.

SYMPTOMS: Nausea, vomiting, flatulence, abdominal pain, cramping and diarrhoea. When the food allergy is associated with other allergies, symptoms may also include a rash, eczema, rhinitis, wheezing, angioedema and occasionally anaphylaxis.

DIAGNOSIS: Unless the reaction occurs immediately after a meal, the allergen may be difficult to identify. Medical diagnoses are usually made with a skin-prick test or a blood test.

FOOD INTOLERANCE

Food intolerance occurs when food is not properly broken down or absorbed. It often comes about as a result of deficiencies in particular enzymes in the gut. Examples of this condition include lactose intolerance (an inability to digest lactose, the sugar in milk), and irritable bowel syndrome. Some people react to the additives in processed food, and the severity of a reaction is often related to the amount of offending substance eaten. Additives are placed in food either to lengthen its shelf-life or to make it more appealing; for example, by enhancing colour, texture or flavour. You are most

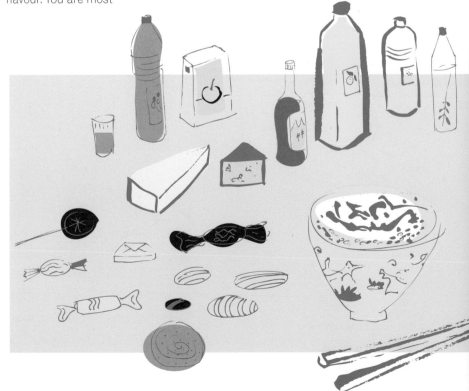

likely to react badly to a food additive if you are already afflicted by some form of allergy, such as asthma or hay fever. The biggest troublemakers are:

◆ Antioxidants, such as ascorbic acid in butter: Used to stop fats and oils from going rancid. Antioxidants can cause rashes, hives and tight chests.

◆ Colorants, such as tartrazine. This is a yellow food colorant that seems to cause the release of histamine, thus exacerbating the symptoms of allergies. Many people think they react to tartrazine but in fact it probably affects only one person in a thousand. Foods containing colorants include fruit juices, soft drinks, cooking oils, and sweets.

◆ Flavour enhancers: These accentuate the natural flavour of foods. The best-known and most controversial is monosodium glutamate (MSG). Foods that contain MSG include oriental meals, dried soup mixes and soy sauce. MSG also occurs naturally in mushrooms and tomatoes. for more information on MSG see www.truthinlabeling.org.

◆ Sodium benzoate: Used as a preservative; for example, to stop fruit juices and soft drinks from spoiling. This substance is thought to create more problems than any other additive.

◆ Sulphur dioxide and sulphites: Used as a preservative or bleach. Sulphiting agents prevent discoloration (for example, of dried fruit and potatoes), and bacterial growth in wine, beer, and some sauces and pickles. They must be sprayed on to fresh produce, and can be found in fruit juices and concentrated soft drinks. Sulphur dioxide and sulphites destroy vitamin B1 and can cause severe reactions, especially in asthmatics. Up to 40 per cent of children with asthma are thought to be sensitive to these substances. Sulphur dioxide and sodium benzoate can cause a scratchy feeling at the back of the throat, and 'tight chests' in those with asthma.

◆ Sweeteners, such as Aspartame. These are used as a sugar substitute in low-calorie foods. Aspartame may cause rashes or hives, dizziness, hallucinations, and headaches. Other symptoms include throat irritation, wheezing, a worsening of eczema, stomach pains, vomiting and diarrhoea.

◆ Tartrazine and foods rich in histamine, such as fish, certain cheeses, cured meats and some alcoholic beverages can cause sneezing, flushing, runny nose, headaches, and wheezing.

◆ MSG can cause headaches, a burning sensation along the back of the neck, chest tightness or pain (especially in asthmatics), nausea, sweating, a sensation of facial pressure and tingling in the limbs, face and head.

DIAGNOSIS: Intolerances are often diagnosed through exclusion diets. However, it is possible to test for food intolerances with a blood test that measures levels of an antibody called IgG. It is important to note, however, that laboratory tests fail to identify many food intolerances.

TREATMENT: The obvious solution to a food allergy or an intolerance is to eliminate the offending food from the diet. In the case of a severe allergy, this is vital. People who react to food additives should endeavour to maintain a diet of fresh, unprocessed foods. Some studies show that up to 40 per cent of people with chronic urticaria improve or even resolve their condition on an additive-free diet.

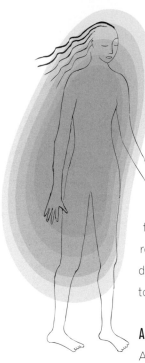

ALLERGIC CONDITIONS

The list of symptoms on page 35 will enable you to pinpoint the conditions that are undermining your health. What follows is a detailed description of each of the allergies and allergy-like disorders mentioned in the chart: what they are, how they come about, who is generally affected and what can be done to treat them. Once you are fully informed, you may well decide to investigate your suspected condition further with an appropriate medical test to confirm or rebut your suspicions. To this end, the following also describes the diagnostic tools that enable allergy sufferers to identify their conditions.

ASTHMA

Asthma is a chronic inflammatory disorder that causes swelling of the airway lining and irritation of the muscle around the airways. This in turn leads to a narrowing of the bronchial passages in the lungs, which affects breathing. Asthma can be severely disabling and has become increasingly prevalent in the developed world: some 3.4 million people use an inhaler on a daily basis.

Inflammation of the airways makes affected individuals very sensitive to all matter that is suspended in the air. There is virtually no limit to the list of airborne triggers that may bring on an asthma attack or awaken asthma symptoms, but the most common trouble-makers in the developed world are indoor allergens. Fifty to 80 per cent of asthmatics are allergic to house-dust mites, 33 to 35 per cent to cats, 10 to 40 per cent to dogs and 10 to 15 per cent to mould. Air pollution is another important trigger, as are certain drugs, stress and the common cold virus. Food allergy is only rarely a cause of asthma (food is implicated in about five per cent of cases), though it is not unusual for an individual to have both asthma and a food allergy in what is known as a multi-system reaction. The link between hay fever and asthma is unclear.

SYMPTOMS: Laboured and noisy breathing; mouth breathing; tightness in the chest; shortness of breath; recurrent episodes of coughing and wheezing; poor concentration; difficulty sleeping.

DIAGNOSIS: Skin-prick test to identify the allergen.

TREATMENT: Antihistamines, topical steroids and other anti-inflammatories, bronchodilators, antileukotrienes.

RHINITIS

Rhinitis is a reaction that occurs in the eyes, nose and throat and is classed as either allergic or non-allergic.

Allergic rhinitis arises when airborne particles or allergens trigger the release of histamine, which in turn causes inflammation and fluid production in the fragile lining of nasal passages, sinuses, and eyelids. The condition is further subdivided into seasonal rhinitis (hayfever), which occurs particularly during the pollen seasons, and perennial rhinitis, which occurs throughout the year and is of primary concern in the context of this book. The most common causes of perennial allergic rhinitis are biological allergens, such as dust mites, mould and pets.

The condition may appear for the first time at any age, though it becomes increasingly common during childhood, and is at its most prevalent among people in their late twenties and early thirties. For some people, the condition dwindles with the passing of years, though in others the condition remains constant throughout their lives, and the disorder may appear for the first time at any age.

Non-allergic rhinitis is otherwise known as sinusitis, and more often than not it follows an infection, such as the common cold. The result is a mucus blockage in the sinuses, which can lead to a secondary infection and a painful swelling of the lining of the nose. Acute sinusitis usually lasts up to ten days, whereas chronic sinusitis can persist for many weeks. Other causes of non-allergic rhinitis include an abnormality in the shape of the nose, nasal polyps and a host of other poorly understood disorders. Triggers include indoor and outdoor pollution, strong smells, temperature fluctuations, atmospheric changes and smoke.

The symptoms of allergic and non-allergic rhinitis are so similar that even experienced doctors have difficulty making a diagnosis. To complicate matters further, there is often some overlap between the conditions. For example, the swollen mucous membranes caused by allergic rhinitis provide the optimum environment for an infection to take root, so at times allergic rhinitis may be an indirect trigger of chronic sinusitis.

SYMPTOMS FOR ALL TYPES OF RHINITIS: Sneezing; blocked nose; mouth-breathing; runny nose; itchy nose, throat, palate, eyes and ears; blocked ears; pale mucous membranes; facial pain; headache; catarrh; poor concentration; difficulty sleeping. Seen more rarely: nasal polyps, dark circles under eyes (caused by increased blood flow near the sinuses), fatigue, voice change, irritating cough, loss or alteration of smell.

DIAGNOSIS: To help doctors differentiate between allergic and non-allergic rhinitis, an otoscope is used, enabling the doctor to look into the nose and the sinuses. If an allergy is suspected, skin-prick tests are performed.

TREATMENT FOR ALLERGIC RHINITIS: The following are prescribed by a doctor either singly or in combination: Antihistamines; topical nasal steroids and eye drops; inhaled medicines; cromolyn sodium; immunotherapy.

TREATMENT FOR NON-ALLERGIC RHINITIS: This may include oral medicines such as decongestants; antibiotics to treat acute bacterial sinusitis and a longer course of antibiotics for chronic sinusitis (sometimes for up to six weeks); surgery to correct the shape of the nose; removal of nasal polyps; nasal steroid sprays or drops, or a short course of steroid tablets to treat an underlying allergy.

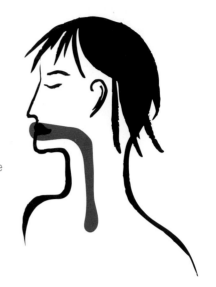

ORAL ALLERGY SYNDROME

Some people with food allergies experience a local tissue reaction on the lips, in the mouth and in the throat, in what is known as Oral Allergy Syndrome (OAS). Fresh fruit and vegetables are the usual triggers; however, some people are allergic to eggs and shellfish. Also, oral allergy usually goes hand-in-hand with pollen allergy, occurring when the immune system mistakes an ingested ingredient for pollen. Reactions characteristically occur within minutes of ingesting the offending food. They are rarely severe and usually vanish fairly quickly.

SYMPTOMS: Localised symptoms include itching of lips, mouth, or pharynx and angioedema of the lips, tongue, palate, and throat. Occasionally blisters may also appear. At its worst, OAS appears as glottic oedema (fluid in the windpipe), usually when the person is allergic to celery. OAS may be manifested in other parts of the body as urticaria, rhinitis, conjunctivitis, asthma, or anaphylaxis (about 2 per cent of people with OAS suffer anaphylactic attacks as a result).

DIAGNOSIS: A thorough medical history, skin-prick test, or blood test to identify the allergen.

TREATMENT: Allergen avoidance; antihistamines; adrenaline (in the event of anaphylaxis); treatment as appropriate for an underlying pollen allergy.

ALLERGIC CONJUNCTIVITIS

This eye condition affects an estimated 6 out of 10 allergy sufferers and is triggered by a range of airborne allergens and irritants from tree, grass and ragweed pollen; flakes of dandruff from animals; medicine applied to the skin; cosmetics; and household chemicals. Seasonal allergic conjunctivitis is usually linked to attacks of hayfever. It is inadvisable to wear contact lenses during an allergic reaction, as this may make symptoms worse or lead to an eye infection.

You may be the only person in your home who spends half the day in tears while everyone else is permanently dry-eyed. This is because a person's risk of mounting an allergic response depends on a series of interrelated factors such as their genetic make up, their state of psychological and physical health, the concentration of the contaminant and the duration and frequency of each exposure.

SYMPTOMS: Red and swollen eyelid membranes; crusting of the eyelids; red, itchy, uncomfortable, watery eyes; runny nose; repeated sneezing.

DIAGNOSIS: Skin-prick test or patch test to identify the allergen.

TREATMENT: Lubricating eye drops (sometimes called artificial tears) to reduce swelling. A cold compress over the eyes may bring relief. Antihistamines in tablet form can reduce itching, redness, swelling and discomfort. Eye drops containing a combination of antihistamine and decongestant are used both to relieve symptoms and prevent them from reappearing, but they should not be used for more than two weeks. Other drugs that have been shown to help itchy, watery eyes and keep symptoms from returning are ketorolac tromethamine (not suitable for people with an allergy to aspirin or ibuprofen or with a bleeding disorder), levocabastine and olopatadine. Steroid eye drops are sometimes used if the allergic conjunctivitis is severe, but patients should discuss side effects with their doctor first.

ECZEMA

Eczema refers to a lesion of the skin, and is used to describe any condition that manifests itself as a red, blistering, oozing, scaly, flaky, itchy or painful rash. It comes from the Greek word for 'boiling over', and affects over 5 million people in the UK and 3 million people in Australia, 10 per cent of whom will have it for life.

TREATMENT: Emollient creams, steroid creams or wet-wrapping. Wet-wrapping is an extremely effective treatment for children with severe eczema, and is particularly useful for breaking the dreaded scratch–itch cycle. (See page 29 for details.) However, it is essential that this treatment be practised under medical supervision, as wet-wrapping infected skin can lead to a very serious condition called eczema herpetiform.

ATOPIC DERMATITIS

This is an allergic skin reaction, otherwise known as atopic eczema, generated from within the body. It is common all over the world, affecting about 10 per cent of infants in developed countries, and there is a strong hereditary element to the condition.

In 75 per cent of children with atopic dermatitis, the symptoms appear before six months of age. Most people grow out of the condition by the age of five, and those who carry it into their teens usually shake it off by their mid-twenties. However, some people are affected throughout their lives, and many of those who grow out of it persist with some degree of contact dermatitis.

In some cases – though not all – there is link between diet and eczema flare-ups. Children in particular may notice a worsening in their condition if they eat certain things. Foods that are most commonly implicated in flare-ups are cow's milk, soy, eggs, fish, wheat and peanuts.

Many people with eczematous skin, and especially children, become caught in the so-called scratch–itch cycle, where an overwhelming need to scratch, especially at night, leads to open sores and localised infection. Some children are affected by atopic eczema so badly that their skin is permanently raw, painful and inflamed. Even in these cases, however, infantile eczema usually improves by the time the child reaches the age of two. (Disability allowance is available for childhood eczema in the UK.)

The number of substances that can cause atopic dermatitis to flare up are virtually limitless. Common triggers include house-dust mites; chemicals; latex; hair and beauty products; cosmetics; and water when the skin is soaked in it for extended periods. Stress and tiredness can be other contributory factors.

SYMPTOMS: The skin rash from atopic dermatitis is often very itchy and sometimes disfiguring. In infancy, the condition tends to manifest as itching, weeping, blistering, crusting skin, appearing mainly on the face and scalp, though patches can appear anywhere. This tends to develop into dry, scaly, thickened and bark-like skin in older children. In teenagers and adults, eczema patches typically occur on the elbow bends, backs of the knees, ankles, wrists, and on the face, neck and upper chest, though any area may be affected. People with latex allergy experience the onset of a rash in the area of contact 24 to 48 hours after exposure, though skin blisters may spread to other areas of the body, too.

DIAGNOSIS: Skin-prick test; blood test.

TREATMENT: External medicines include corticosteroid (cortisone) creams or ointments, although some people are allergic to these; tar creams; antihistamines taken in tablet form to control the itching; oral antibiotics to treat secondary infection; ultraviolet light therapy for severe cases; sedative antihistamines when itching interrupts sleep; wet-wrapping (see opposite). Cortisone in pill form should be avoided if possible, though it may be prescribed if other medication fails. Sufferers should avoid smallpox vaccination; rough, scratchy or tight clothing and woollens; rapid changes of temperature; any activity that provokes sweating. Creams and lotions can bring relief.

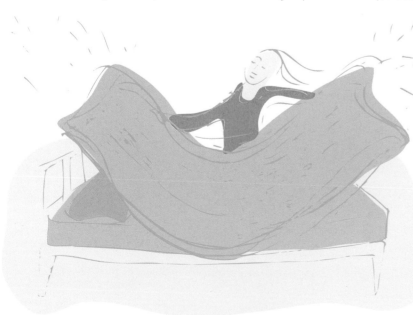

WET-WRAPPING

The principle behind wet-wrapping is to moisturise the child's body then send him or her to bed with limbs and torso enveloped in two layers of bandage, one wet and one dry, to ensure that much of the moisture remains close to the body. Emollients can be used alone or in conjunction with steroid creams (though the two must be applied at least 20 minutes apart), and a pair of cotton pyjamas should be worn on top to prevent the cream rubbing off onto sheets. Wet-wrapping must always be carried out under medical supervision

ALLERGIC CONTACT DERMATITIS

When a substance touches the skin, penetrates the surface and triggers a response from the part of the immune system located in the uppermost layer, the resulting eczema is known as allergic contact dermatitis (symptoms are similar for non-allergic contact dermatitis, a condition that arises when the immune system is not involved in the skin's response to an irritant).

Allergic contact dermatitis is a condition that can develop at any stage in life as a direct result of skin sensitisation. It happens when a usually harmless substance suddenly triggers an aggressive skin reaction, and once it has developed, contact allergy is a lifelong condition. Exposing the skin to even a minute quantity of the offending substance is liable to trigger a response, even years after the initial reaction. Common triggers include household chemicals; cosmetics and beauty products; natural and synthetic fragrances; materials used in home construction.

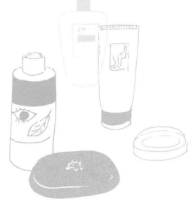

SYMPTOMS: The first sign of contact dermatitis is often itchy, flushed skin with tiny fluid-filled blisters and moist patches. Symptoms are often delayed, and the rash may appear even a week after contact with the offending substance. As the condition becomes more chronic, dryness and scales usually develop and may become permanent. Once an area has become sensitised, complete avoidance is the only solution, as exposure to the allergen even years later will immediately trigger a rash.

DIAGNOSIS: Patch testing.

TREATMENT: External medications include corticosteroid (cortisone) creams or ointments (some people are allergic to these) and tar creams. Avoid internally administered cortisone, though it may be prescribed if other medicine fails. Sufferers should avoid rough, scratchy or tight clothing and woollens, rapid changes of temperature and any activity that provokes sweating. Creams and lotions can bring relief.

URTICARIA (CHRONIC HIVES OR NETTLE RASH)

This is a very distressing condition that is sometimes linked to an allergy. In most people, nettle rash lasts only a few weeks, and in these cases a viral infection may be the underlying cause. Nettle rash lasting more than six weeks is classified as chronic, and in only about 30 per cent of cases are doctors able to identify a cause, such as an underlying disease (perhaps a thyroid, liver, or sinus problems), an allergic reaction to a drug, insect or food or a reaction to a food additive. For the remaining 70 per cent of cases, doctors usually blame the disease on an overactive immune system and a precise cause or cure might never be found.

SYMPTOMS: Nettle rash manifests itself as a red or pink rash. It varies in shape, from a collection of small bumps to blotchy or streaky areas; it is very itchy and appears at irregular intervals, later disappearing without a trace. When nettle rash is caused by an allergic reaction, it usually breaks out within one hour of exposure to the allergen.

An underlying food allergy may be the cause of nettle rash if the condition is accompanied by the following symptoms: indigestion, fullness and bloating; abdominal pain, diarrhoea and irritable-bowel-like symptoms; acute sneezing attacks and rhinitis; acute asthma attacks with no obvious cause; itching of the palms, feet and scalp.

DIAGNOSIS: A careful medical history is most useful. Laboratory tests are generally not helpful, though a skin-prick test may yield useful results if the patient relates symptoms to the ingestion of a particular type of food.

TREATMENT: Where there is an underlying disease or allergy, this should be treated. Where there is no known cause for the condition, the best that can be done is to prevent the nettle rash from breaking out. Antihistamines constitute the main treatment. If these do not work, a doctor may prescribe a short course of steroid-type pills to clear the rash, followed by long-term antihistamines to maintain the effect.

PERSISTENT NETTLE RASH
In half the cases of nettle rash, the condition spontaneously resolves in about six months, but in 20 per cent of cases it is still present after 20 years. Unfortunately, there's no cure, but when the condition is persistent, patients can learn strategies to prevent the rash from appearing in the first place.

ANGIOEDEMA

This condition often accompanies nettle rash, and is caused by small blood vessels deep in the skin or gut leaking liquid through their walls, causing a swelling. Like nettle rash, angioedema may result from an allergy, though more often than not it occurs without apparent cause. The condition can be acute, lasting from a few minutes to a few days, or chronic, meaning that it recurs for years. Acute symptoms may be triggered by an allergy to drugs, food or latex. Occasionally chronic recurrent angioedema results from a shortage or abnormality of a blood protein called C1 inhibitor. The cause is more often unknown.

SYMPTOMS: Swelling can be very prominent and is particularly common in the lips and other parts of the mouth and throat, the eyelids, genitals, hands and feet. At worst, the tongue becomes so swollen that speech is impeded. The condition is life-threatening if swelling in the throat makes breathing difficult (Angioedema is a feature of anaphylaxis.) Fortunately this happens only rarely.

DIAGNOSIS: The same as for urticaria.

TREATMENT: Antihistamines, adrenaline inhalers or injections if symptoms include swelling in the mouth or throat.

PHOTOSENSITIVITY

Photosensitive individuals usually react on a bright summer's day though reactions can occur in winter too. Very sensitive subjects may even be affected by fluorescent lamps indoors. Some people affected by this condition are sensitive to just one kind of sunlight, while others react to a combination of UV radiation. The most common photosensitivity is to UVA. In some cases, the cause of photosensitivity is never discovered. It might be brought on by a metabolic disorder such as Porphyria, or an autoimmune disease such as Lupus Erythematosus.

Common triggers include cosmetics and medications applied to the skin. Some topical treatments are structurally altered by UV light, provoking the skin in susceptible people to produce antibodies in what is known as a photoallergic reaction. Troublemakers include synthetic musk, sandalwood oil and bergamot oil. Medicines (especially antihistamines, pain relievers and some antibiotics, including the tetracyclines and the sulphonamides) can also trigger reactions.

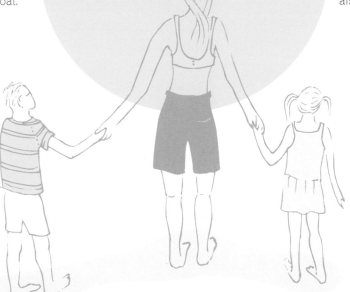

SYMPTOMS: Acute effects from short-term exposure include exaggerated sunburned-like skin; eye burn; mild allergic reactions such as hives; abnormal reddening of the skin; and eczema-like rashes. Symptoms can appear 20 seconds after sun exposure, producing eczema-like conditions that can spread to non-exposed parts of the body. Chronic effects from long-term exposure include premature skin ageing; stronger allergic skin reactions; cataracts; blood vessel damage; a weakened immune system; skin cancer.

DIAGNOSIS: Photosensitivity can be confirmed by a Phototest, in which artificial light from different sources is shone on small areas of the skin to see whether the rash can be reproduced, or if sunburn occurs more easily than expected. If the condition is induced by contact with a chemical substance, adhesive patches containing known photosensitising materials are applied to the upper back, removed after two days, and light is shone on the area. The reaction is observed two days later.

TREATMENT: Photosensitivity may clear up when an underlying disease is treated or a known trigger is avoided. Protecting the skin from sunlight is also key. This can be achieved by wearing high-factor sunscreens in all weather, even in the car or house (UVA can pass through glass), paying special attention to sensitive areas such as lips. Sunscreens come in two types: chemical sunscreens that absorb sunlight, and physical sunblocks (zinc and titanium dioxide), which reflect sunlight. The second type is messy to apply but is better for people with very sensitive skin, or those with allergies to the chemicals in sunscreens. Wear densely woven clothing; apply UV-absorbing film to windows at home or in the car. If the sensitivity is severe and disabling, consider wearing a mask to cover the face for trips outside (clear ones are available). Favour ordinary tungsten light bulbs over unguarded fluorescent lamps. It is perfectly safe to watch television.

DERMATITIS HERPETIFORMIS

This type of rash is caused by a gluten sensitivity that also affects the small intestine (see 'Coeliac disease' below). But it is not just gluten in the diet that causes dermatitis herpetiformis to flare up in affected individuals. Other triggers include iodides (some iodine is needed in the diet); kelp; shellfish; non-steroidal anti-inflammatory agents such as aspirin; stress; some chemicals.

SYMPTOMS: An itchy skin rash that consists of red raised patches and small blisters, commonly occurring on the elbows, buttocks and knees, though any area of the body may be affected.

DIAGNOSIS: A skin biopsy followed by a test known as immunofluorescence, which reveals antibodies specific to the condition.

TREATMENT: A gluten-free (GF) diet sometimes accompanied by drugs to suppress the blisters. The drugs most commonly used are either a sulphone (Dapsone) or a sulphonamide (Sulphapyradine). In about 85 per cent of cases, at least a year on a strict gluten-free diet is needed before this skin condition is resolved.

COELIAC DISEASE

This is a lifelong inflammatory condition of the intestinal tract that affects the small intestine in genetically susceptible individuals. It is caused by gluten, a protein in wheat, and similar proteins in rye, barley and oats. In a coeliac, gluten damages the lining of the small intestine, which greatly reduces the gut's ability to absorb adequate nutrients from food. Coeliac disease affects thousands of people across the globe. Symptoms appear in babies after weaning on to gluten-containing solids.

SYMPTOMS:

In infants: Diarrhoea with bulky, pale, offensive-smelling stools; vomiting; miserable disposition; failure to thrive.

In adults: Vomiting, diarrhoea, weight loss, tiredness, lethargy, breathlessness. Most people experience only a few of these symptoms and some have no obvious symptoms.

DIAGNOSIS: An intestinal biopsy, usually under mild sedation.

TREATMENT: A strict gluten-free diet resolves symptoms, though sufferers must adhere to this eating regime permanently to avoid a recurrence of their illness.

ANAPHYLAXIS

An anaphylactic attack is very rapid and involves organ systems throughout the body. Immediate medical attention is required. Common causes include certain foods and types of medicine, especially penicillin; anaesthetic drugs; intravenous infusion liquids; certain injected drugs (for example, blood clot-busting drugs used after heart attacks); some substances injected during X-rays.

People with a food allergy often notice the effect of anaphylaxis in seconds, and their life may be in jeopardy within a few minutes. However, in some instances, a serious reaction can take much longer to start (an hour or more). If the onset of symptoms coincides with strenuous exercise, the attack is often ascribed to Food-Related Exercise-induced Anaphylaxis. Such an attack can occur up to 24 hours after ingesting an allergenic food. Foods likely to cause a reaction are nuts, shellfish, sesame, soy, eggs, milk, fruit and (rarely) spices. Restaurant food for allergic individuals should be prepared with separate utensils to avoid cross-contamination.

ADRENALINE JABS

People at risk of anaphylaxis, along with family members, should be trained to administer adrenaline in an emergency. The medication should be carried by the at-risk individual at all times in a pre-loaded injection kit. The kit must be kept in a clearly marked robust pouch or case within easy reach, protected from direct sunlight and high temperatures and replaced before the expiry date.

In people with latex allergy, anaphylaxis may occur after exposure to rubber latex items. Certain foods related to the rubber tree (*Hevea brasiliensis*) can also trigger a reaction insensitive individuals. Insect stings, especially bee or wasp stings, are also known to induce anaphylaxis. (See page 49.) However, a substantial proportion of attacks have no known trigger.

People at risk of anaphylaxis should always wear an anaphylactic warning bracelet or pendant, and carry adrenaline, a hormone produced naturally by the body, in a pre-loaded injection kit. This should be protected from direct sunlight and high temperatures.

SYMPTOMS: An itchy nettle rash (urticaria, hives); swelling (angioedema) in the throat, causing difficulty in swallowing or breathing; asthma symptoms; vomiting; cramping stomach pain; diarrhoea; a tingling feeling in the lips or mouth (if the cause was a food); faintness and unconsciousness due to very low blood pressure (anaphylactic shock). People who are allergic to insect bites may notice a rash in parts of their body that were not stung. A few people have a second wave of anaphylaxis after treatment, so anyone who experiences a serious anaphylactic reaction should be observed medically for about six hours or overnight.

DIAGNOSIS: Blood test.

TREATMENT: It may be difficult to decide if the cause of symptoms is anaphylaxis, fainting for an unrelated reason, or a panic attack. If in doubt, a thorough medical investigation should be pursued. A highly effective and fast-acting treatment for true anaphylaxis is an injection of adrenaline, which should be administered before the patient falls unconscious. (See also page 40.)

Anaphylaxis is sometimes mild, with no immediate need for treatment. However, an apparently mild attack may develop into a life-threatening condition, so medical help should always be sought. The fact that previous anaphylactic attacks have been mild does not guarantee that they will be minor in the future.

ALLERGY SYMPTOMS

This list describes the range of symptoms that may be triggered by an allergy, and is intended as a guide to likely diagnoses. However, it must be stressed that conventional medical tests should be sought to confirm or refute self-diagnosis. An asterisk is used to signify that a symptom – for example, the chest tightness of asthma – might actually be caused by another condition, such as urticaria.

RESPIRATORY SYSTEM

Breathlessness: asthma; coeliac disease

Tightness in the chest: asthma; food intolerance*; urticaria*

Shortness of breath: asthma; urticaria*

Wheezing: asthma; food allergy* or intolerance*

Coughing: asthma; rhinitis

Mouth-breathing: asthma; rhinitis

Swelling in throat or difficulty swallowing: anaphylaxis; angioedema; oral allergy syndrome

Glottic oedema (fluid in the windpipe): oral allergy syndrome

EARS

Itchy ears: food allergy*; rhinitis

Blocked ears: food allergy*; rhinitis

NOSE

Runny nose: conjunctivitis; food intolerance; rhinitis

Sneezing: conjunctivitis; food allergy* or intolerance*; rhinitis; urticaria

Blocked nose: food allergy*; rhinitis

Itchy nose: food allergy*; rhinitis

Catarrh: rhinitis

Nasal polyps: rhinitis

Loss/alteration of smell: rhinitis

Upward rubbing in children: asthma; conjunctivitis; rhinitis

EYES

Red, swollen and watery eyes: conjunctivitis

Red and swollen eyelids: conjunctivitis

Itchy eyes: conjunctivitis; food allergy*; rhinitis

Dark circles: rhinitis

Eye-burn: photosensitivity

(In small children, dark lines known as Denny's lines are a more common symptom.)

MOUTH

Itching of lips, mouth or pharynx: oral allergy syndrome

Swelling of the lips, tongue, palate and throat: oral allergy syndrome

Blisters in mouth: oral allergy syndrome

Itchy palate: food allergy*; rhinitis

Tingling in lips and mouth: anaphylaxis

Mouth-breathing and snoring: rhinitis

SKIN

Itchy, weeping, blistering or crusting: eczema (particularly atopic dermatitis); food allergy*; photosensitivity

Fluid-filled blisters and moist patches: eczema (particularly allergic contact dermatitis)

Flushed appearance: eczema; food intolerance

Dry skin and scales: allergic contact dermatitis

Red/pink rash, collection of small bumps with blotches or streaky areas: photosensitivity; urticaria

General itchy rash: allergic contact dermatitis; atopic dermatitis; dermatitis herpetiformis; photosensitivity; urticaria

Itchy palms, feet and scalp: urticaria

Itchy elbows, buttocks and knees: dermatitis herpetiformis

Prominent swelling, particularly on lips and other parts of mouth, throat, eyelids, genitals, hands and feet: angioedema; food allergy*

Sunburned-appearance: photosensitivity

Sweating: food intolerance

DIGESTIVE SYSTEM

Indigestion, fullness, bloating, flatulence, abdominal pain, cramping, diarrhoea: anaphylaxis; food allergy; latex allergy*; urticaria*

Nausea, vomiting: anaphylaxis; coeliac disease; food allergy or intolerance

Weight loss: coeliac disease

OTHER

Face pain: food allergy*; rhinitis

Pale mucous membranes: rhinitis

Difficulty sleeping: asthma; eczema; rhinitis

Poor concentration: asthma; coeliac disease; rhinitis

Headache: food intolerance

Lethargy: coeliac disease

Feeling of faintness: anaphylaxis

Unconsciousness: anaphylaxis

Tingling in limbs, face or head: food intolerance

Hallucinations: food intolerance

Diagnosis

The aim of allergy testing is to identify the specific substance causing an allergy. In a non-allergic person, there should be no response to the allergen; a positive test most often indicates an allergy to the substance in question. However, any professional interpreting a skin, blood or patch test must view the results in light of the patient's medical history, and no test should be read in isolation.

SKIN-PRICK TESTING

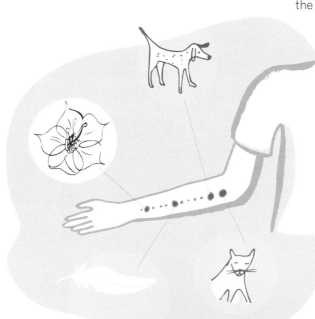

This is the most commonly used allergy test and is an effective test for allergic conjunctivitis, allergic rhinitis, asthma, penicillin allergy and insect-bite allergies. It involves placing one drop of each suspected substance on the skin (usually on the lower inner arm), pricking or scratching the skin with a lancet so the allergen is introduced under the surface, then observing any reactions. Between three and 25 potential allergens can be tested at once, each of which is coded on the patient's skin. Reliable skin testing for food allergy requires the use of fresh food and high-quality skin-testing products. False negative reactions often occur.

If the individual has bad eczema on the forearm, the test is usually performed on the back. Anyone who has experienced an anaphylactic attack should *not* submit to a skin-prick test, as the experiment itself may trigger a life-threatening reaction. An allergy will show up within a few minutes as a small itchy weal with a raised edge, surrounded by an inflamed area. The weal will appear within 20 minutes and will fade usually within an hour. Cough medicine and some antidepressants can interfere with results, so patients should avoid taking these for about five days prior to the test. The antihistamine Hismanal (Astemizole) should be stopped six weeks prior to the test.

PATCH TESTING

This test is performed in cases where contact dermatitis is suspected. The potential allergens are prepared in white soft paraffin and spread onto small metallic discs. These are then placed on the skin (usually on the back) and stuck down with hypoallergenic tape. The patches are removed after 48 hours, the skin is examined and any redness or swellings are noted. The skin is re-examined after another 48 hours for any remaining local redness or swelling. Interpreting the results of a patch test is usually left to specialist dermatologists.

Eczema symptoms need to be brought under control before patch testing can be carried out or the results will be unreliable. Steroid creams should not be used for three to four weeks before testing, as these may suppress the allergic response.

UNPREDICTABLE RESULTS

One drawback of skin-prick tests is that a positive reaction will occur even in people who are not allergic if the dose of an allergen is excessive. Also, a negative response to a given allergen usually indicates that the patient is not sensitive to that allergen, but not always; for example, the skin of some elderly people may not be capable of reacting.

BLOOD TESTING

This is an effective test for individuals at risk of an anaphylactic reaction; those with extensive eczema for whom skin-prick testing is impractical; and those who cannot stop taking antihistamine medication because their allergy symptoms are so severe.

The blood test is called UniCAP (a third generation RAST – radioallergosorbent – test) and measures the amount of specific IgE produced by the immune system and circulating in the blood. Results are classed from 0 to 6 depending on the individual's sensitivity to an allergen (0 = no sensitivity, 4–6 = extreme sensitivity).

OTHER TESTS

◆ Elimination tests: Suspected food allergens are eliminated for several weeks then gradually reintroduced one at a time while the person is observed for signs of an allergic reaction. For reliable results, placebos (non-food substances) should be included in the experiment.

◆ Skin biopsy: Used to diagnose dermatitis herpetiformis.

◆ Intestinal biopsy: Used to diagnose coeliac disease.

◆ Otoscope: Used for internal examination of the nose and sinuses when doctors cannot readily distinguish between allergic and non-allergic rhinitis.

◆ Phototest: Used to diagnose photosensitivity.

◆ Alternative tests include Applied Kinesiology (measures muscle strength); Auricular Cardiac Reflex Method (measures strongest pulse at the wrist); Hair Analysis (tests for a range of medical problems); Leukocytotoxic Tests (white blood cells are mixed with suspected allergen and observed under a microscope); Neutralisation–Provocation Testing (neutralised allergen drops are placed under the tongue); Vega Testing (measures the electromagnetic fields produced by the person).

Treatments

Three general approaches to allergy treatment are taken by practitioners of conventional medicine: allergen avoidance, prescribed medicine to relieve and control symptoms, and a programme of allergy injections (immunotherapy). Avoidance is discussed in detail in the Solutions chapter. Here, information on the other two treatment options are reviewed.

PRESCRIBED MEDICINES

These provide effective relief from the symptoms of allergy but do not afford a cure. Treatments should be reviewed annually, unless they are ineffective, in which case the prescribing doctor should be consulted right away.

ANTIHISTAMINES

These work by blocking histamine, the major chemical released by the body when it is exposed to an allergen. They relieve the symptoms of asthma, allergic rhinitis, allergic conjunctivitis, atopic dermatitis, urticaria and angioedema but do not treat chronic inflammation. The new, non-sedating antihistamines are preferable to the older type. Antihistamines can be taken in tablet or liquid form, or as eye drops or nasal sprays. They are often prescribed in combination with other treatments.

ANTILEUKOTRIENES

Leukotrienes are another class of chemical released during an allergic reaction. Antileukotrienes widen the airways to relieve symptoms in asthmatics.

DECONGESTANTS

Oral or nasal decongestants cause a narrowing of small blood vessels in the nasal membranes, thus reducing blood flow to inflamed tissues. This helps to relieve symptoms of allergic rhinitis, such as swelling, excess secretions, a blocked nose and painful sinuses. Non-prescription decongestant nose drops and sprays should not be used for more than a couple of days as they can damage the tissues of the nose and cause aggravation of symptoms, a condition known as rhinitis medicamentosa. Oral decongestants are absorbed into the bloodstream and can interact in an adverse way with other medicines, such as prescription antidepressants, drugs for high blood pressure and medicines for certain heart problems.

BRONCHODILATORS

These drugs are used by asthmatics to relieve the spasm in the airways caused by allergen exposure, and thereby ease breathing. They are usually prescribed as inhalers, and come in two varieties: short-acting, to be used whenever breathing feels uncomfortable; long-acting, which last 12 hours, to be used daily or twice daily to prevent the airways from narrowing. If bronchodilators are used more than four or five times a week on a regular basis, they should be taken in conjunction with an anti-inflammatory drug.

ANTI-INFLAMMATORY MEDICINES

The main anti-inflammatory drugs are corticosteroids, not to be confused with the anabolic steroids used by body builders. Corticosteroids prevent the body from making the chemical messengers called cytokines that prolong the tissue inflammation that is triggered by contact with an allergen. Corticosteroids are, therefore, used to treat the long-term inflammation that characterises chronic conditions such as allergic eczema, asthma, allergic rhinitis and hayfever. They are available as nose sprays (for allergic rhinitis and hayfever); eye drops (for allergic rhinitis, hayfever and allergic conjunctivitis); inhaled aerosols (for asthma); creams or ointments (for atopic dermatitis and allergic contact dermatitis). Corticosteroids are safest taken as inhalers and sprays because they are poorly absorbed into the bloodstream in these forms. Side effects can occur when they are taken as pills or skin treatments. These include reddening and swelling of the face, permanent thinning of the skin, muscle weakness, peptic ulcers, osteoporosis, cataracts in the eye and reduced growth rate in children.

ALLERGIC DRUGS

These drugs are beneficial in preventing allergy symptoms and because they have very few side effects they are often prescribed for children. They act locally in the nasal or conjunctival lining to inhibit the release of histamine and other allergy-related chemicals from cells in the body. However, they are not particularly potent and are therefore useful only for treating mild to moderate allergic diseases. To be effective, they must be taken before a sensitive individual comes into contact with an allergen. So hayfever sufferers should use them throughout the pollen season. The most commonly used allergic drugs are sodium cromoglycate and nedocromil sodium. (Children with asthma are not advised to use nedocromil sodium without first seeking a doctor's advice.) These are available without a prescription as eye drops to treat allergic rhinitis, hayfever and allergic conjunctivitis, and as a nasal spray to treat allergic rhinitis and hayfever. They take a few days to start working and need to be re-applied frequently (often four times daily).

ADRENALINE

A single adrenaline injection is the most successful treatment for anaphylactic reactions (that is, acute, severe allergic reactions). The drug effectively neutralises all the effects on the body of the sudden release into the bloodstream of histamine and leukotrienes.

The preferable injection site is the muscle on the outer side of the thigh. (For further information on this drug, see page 34.)

PETS WITH ALLERGIES

Animals react to many of the same allergens as humans, such as dust mites, airborne moulds, penicillin, grasses and fleas. Some even react to humans.

Symptoms associated with pet atopic dermatitis include itching, scratching, chewing and biting, as well as sore feet, red ears, bottom rubbing and an unpleasant musty skin odour. Contact allergies are commonly triggered by synthetic fabrics, washing powders and pesticides, and symptoms tend to appear as inflamed patches on the stomach, legs and feet. When pets suffer from a skin allergy, they often lick and gnaw their feet. Special booties can be bought to protect dogs' paws if grass is the allergen, which it often is.

The latest research suggests food allergies and intolerances are also fairly common among pets, especially an allergy to yeast, beef and chicken – ingredients found in many commercial food preparations. Symptoms include colitis, weight loss and continual diarrhoea, which at its most severe can cause a pet's tail to rot away. Usually, symptoms clear up after a change of diet.

IMMUNOTHERAPY

Immunotherapy is an established treatment for certain severe allergies. The treatment is carried out by giving increasing doses of purified allergen (usually under the skin of the upper arm) until an allergic person can tolerate allergen exposure without developing major symptoms (though the allergy is not cured).

Immunotherapy programmes require commitment from the patient. Injections are given once a week for the first three months, then once every other week for up to three years. After each injection, the patient is asked to wait in the clinic for an hour so that any serious side effects can be treated quickly.

Allergies that can be treated with immunotherapy are life-threatening reactions to wasp or bee stings; severe hayfever (treatment occurs out of the pollen season); severe animal allergy. Allergies that cannot be treated by immunotherapy include eczema, urticaria, food allergy and (usually) asthma. Respiratory problems associated with asthma may be exacerbated by allergy injections. Exceptions are made if asthma occurs only during the pollen season, or if asthma is combined with a life-threatening reaction to insect stings. In such cases, it is essential for asthma symptoms to be under control throughout the treatment. Immunotherapy treatment is given to children whose asthma is related to allergies from house dust, cat dander, grass pollen and mould. Otherwise, it is not recommended.

WHEN A COUGH IS NOT A COLD
People with allergy symptoms may at first suspect that they have a common cold. It is important to see a doctor about any respiratory illness that lasts more than a couple of weeks. Identifying the causal allergen is the key to taking control of an allergy.

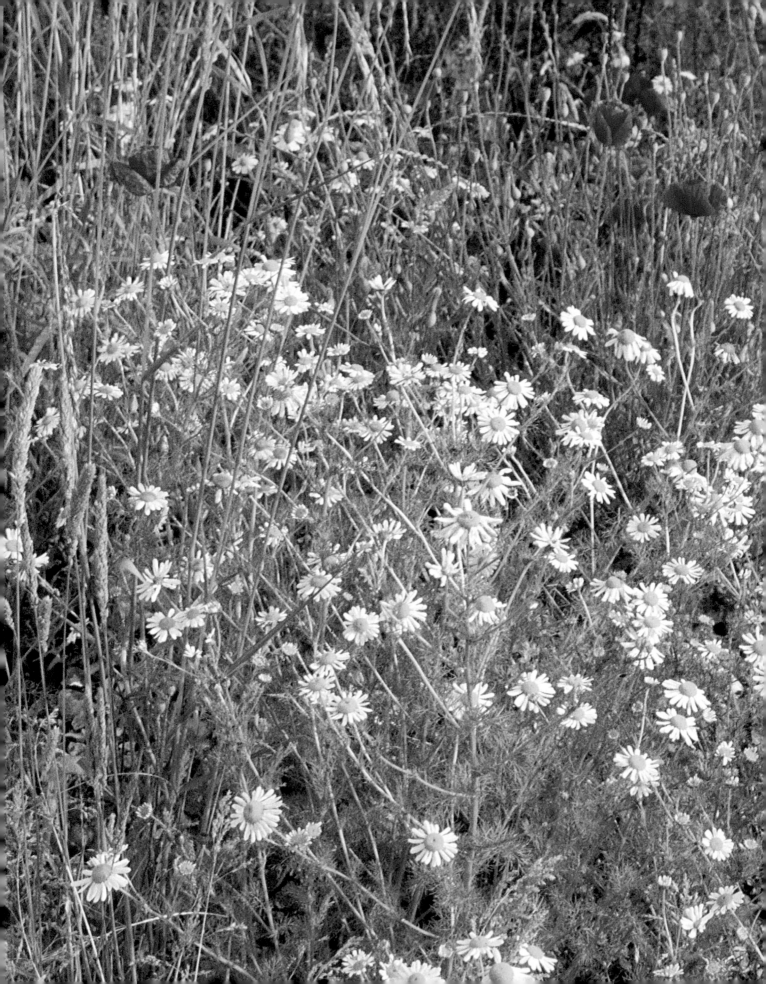

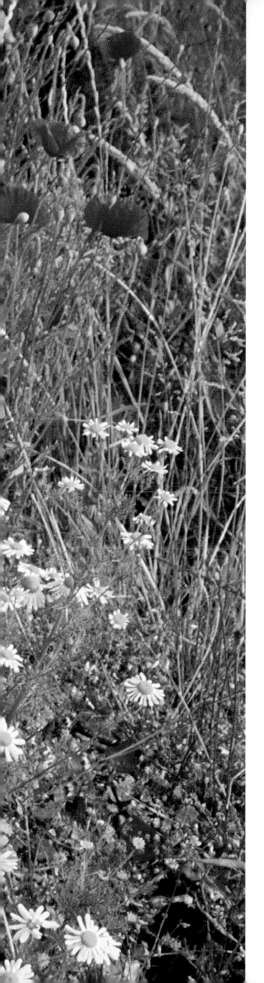

causes and triggers

The average home is a minefield of materials that can provoke abnormal immunological responses in the people living in it. The particles and substances responsible for these responses can be divided into two types: allergens, which trigger true allergies, and irritants, which provoke allergy-like responses. Doctors tend to draw crisp lines between allergens and irritants, but if you happen to be affected by household substances or particles in a way that resembles an allergy, these medical distinctions become irrelevant. The way one person reacts to an irritant is often identical to the way another reacts to an allergen, and both afflicted individuals share a pressing need to identify and then avoid the triggers of their symptoms.

If an indoor substance or particle provokes an abnormal reaction of any kind – whether manifested as an allergy, an intolerance or an irritation – it is treated as a topic of interest here.

Common indoor allergens

Few people realise just how much environmental debris is carried in household dust – from skin particles, clothing fibres, furniture fabric and paint shavings, to soil, chemical residues, dead insects and dust mite particles. House-dust mites are probably the best-studied source of all indoor allergens, and with good reason: they are the single most important cause of allergic symptoms in the home. Knowing how they multiply makes it easier to guard against them.

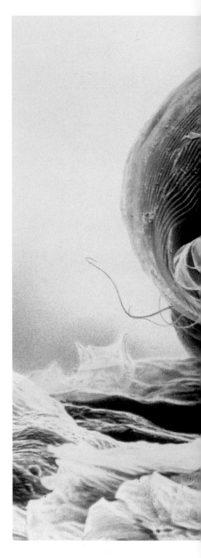

Mattresses and bedding offer perfect living conditions for dust mites. Humans provide moisture through night-time perspiration and a rich, dependable supply of food comes in the form of dead skin flakes.

DUST MITES

Studies in different communities around the world have shown that up to 85 per cent of people with allergic asthma, along with five to 30 per cent of the non-asthmatic population, react to dust mites.

Many modern homes create the ideal conditions in which mites flourish. Central heating provides the warmth they crave and airtight buildings ensure no lack of water molecules trapped indoors.

A typical double mattress hosts up to 2 million mites and contains mite droppings to the tune of several pounds.

And as we spend one third of our lives in bed, this means hours of close contact with copious quantities of potent allergen.

The microscopic mites are harmless enough in themselves – they neither bite nor sting – however, when they defecate, allergy sufferers certainly know about it, as each mite dropping contains sufficient quantities of allergen to trigger asthma, allergic rhinitis and conjunctivitis. One of the main problems with dust mites is that they are so tiny (measuring 0.3mm) and their droppings so minuscule (10 to

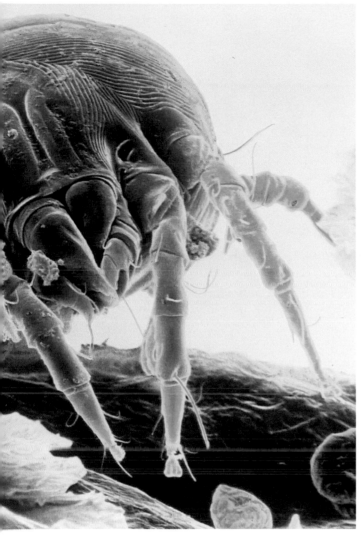

14 microns in size), that it takes minimal disturbance for the allergen to become airborne. Air concentrations in disturbed rooms can be more than a thousand times higher than those observed in undisturbed environments. And once the allergen is circulating in the air, it is easily inhaled into the lungs, where it can precipitate an allergic reaction.

At worst, exposure to mite droppings can trigger an acute asthma attack; when the allergen comes into contact with skin, it can cause eczema. But it is not just those people with an established allergy who should be concerned: there is compelling evidence to suggest that when mite populations reach significant levels, exposure to the allergen can bring about sensitisation in an otherwise healthy individual. This is particularly true of infants. Studies show that the risk of mite-sensitised children developing asthma approximately doubles for every doubling of the level of exposure to mite allergens.

A major obstacle to mite eradication is the speed and efficiency with which they breed, factors that make it virtually impossible to eliminate an entire population from the home. Each mite lives for four months only, but in that time it produces around 200 times its own weight in droppings and lays around 80 eggs. And it is not just our beds that are infested: mites are adaptable little critters, happy to whoop it up in all soft furnishings, from sofas and carpets (there are an estimated 100,000 of them in every square metre of carpet), to curtains and furry toys.

The dust mite is related to spiders and ticks, and in a typical home several species live side by side in perfect harmony. Despite their subtle differences, nearly all species of mite share a common definition of nirvana: a climate that hovers around 25°C with a relative humidity of between 70 and 80 per cent.

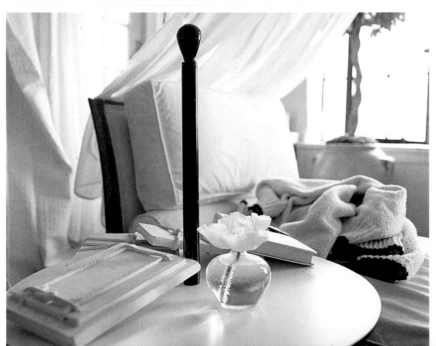

PETS

Domestic animals are the second most prevalent cause of indoor allergic reactions. In the western world, more than 50 per cent of children with allergic asthma are sensitised to allergens of cats, and 40 per cent to dogs. Yet, despite these figures, over half the homes in many developed countries have at least one pet. There is a strong link between the presence of carpeting and high allergen levels.

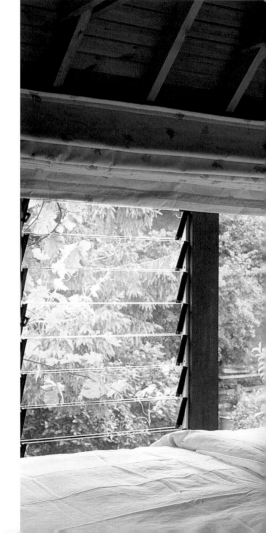

CATS

Cats create the biggest problem. The allergen *Felix domesticus 1* (Fel d1) is found in saliva, dead skin cells and fur (dander). It is spread over the coat as the cat washes and it then dries on the fur. Particles containing allergen are often very fine (less than 0.2 microns in diameter, which means you would get 4.8 million of them in a full stop), so they float into the air as the animal moves. They remain airborne for many hours and are easily inhaled. Much of the allergen never falls to the ground but instead sticks to walls and ceilings by electrostatic forces. Cat allergen may be found on walls and ceilings many months – or even years – after the animal has left the house. They may also be brought into the house on second-hand furniture or transferred from house to house on a visitor's clothes.

BELOW If you are sensitive to animal allergens, your symptoms will certainly worsen if you allow pets to settle on the bed.

DOGS

Dog allergen (Can f1) is mostly found in saliva and dander. Particle size tends to be larger than for cats and so remains airborne for less time.

OTHER ANIMALS

Smaller domestic animals, such as guinea pigs and hamsters, produce allergens in their urine, which is then distributed in their bedding. These allergens become airborne when the animal scurries around in its cage. Budgerigars and parrots are another common cause of allergic reactions, the offending allergens emanating from their feathers.

MOULD, FUNGI, AND SPORES

All homes, if examined closely enough, reveal some mould; however, problems arise only when a building is damp. Rising damp in old buildings and homes with structural faults, and condensation in new, airtight buildings, provide ideal conditions in which fungal life may flourish.

Not only does mould look unpleasant: its spores cause wheezing in children, and 20 per cent of youngsters with allergic asthma are sensitive to mould. There are also links between household mould and fever in children, and high blood pressure and breathlessness in adults.

It is the airborne mould spores that produce allergic and asthmatic reactions among sensitive individuals. Each mould can produce millions of these microscopic seed-like spores, which float in the air and are inhaled. Symptoms tend to be worse on damp days. Mould grows inside damp mattresses, which can be a problem when children wet the bed. In general, homes with mould problems are also likely to have high dust mite levels.

It is often easy to tell if a home has a dampness problem because mould tends to appear as moist patches on the walls, or black, green, blue, or brown patches on window frames, walls, and in bathrooms and kitchens (particularly around refrigerator door seals and shower curtains). However, at times the fungal growth is less obvious and may be visible only as a tiny area of dark pinpoints, which are actually the fruiting bodies releasing large numbers of microscopic spores. The more cunning fungi hide their spores beneath wallpaper and in the soil of house plants. The water reservoirs of dehumidifiers can be another breeding ground for mould if they are not emptied, cleaned and dried daily.

VENTILATION

An individual's exposure to indoor allergens is directly related to the amount of moisture that builds up around them, as constant high humidity encourages dust mites to breed and mould to grow. A household of four people produces up to 12 litres of water vapour daily through perspiration, breathing, bathing, cooking and drying clothes.

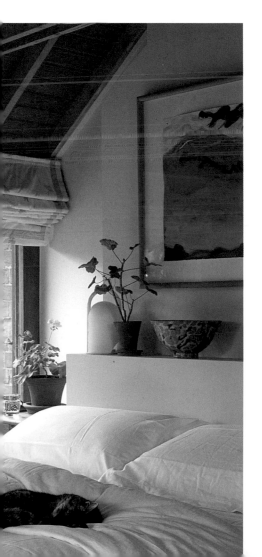

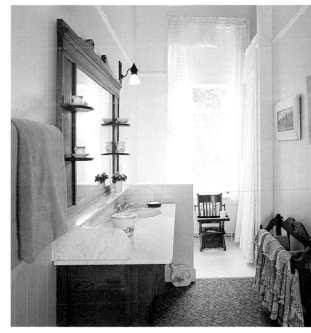

BELOW A damp bathroom is a magnet for allergy-triggering mould. If you have a window, open it; if not, install an extractor fan.

ANT STINGS

In Australia, ant stings can produce life-threatening allergies. The worst offender is a 12mm-long ant called a jumper or hopper ant. This ant is responsible for 90 per cent of serious reactions and is found all over Australia, though most reported cases of severe reactions are from Tasmania and south-eastern Australia. The jumper drops from trees and clothes lines and multiple stings from a number of ants are common. Though the bull ant (2.5cm long) is less agressive than the jumper, it too causes serious allergies.

COCKROACHES

Cockroaches are often associated with crowded cities and tropical climates (and indeed, they are indigenous to the southern United States and Australia); however, these household pests have crossed all continental borders and thrive in much cooler climates, too, courtesy of central heating systems.

Between 5 and 10 per cent of people in Europe are sensitised to cockroach allergen and a far higher percentage of asthmatics test positive to cockroach allergen. An American study found that asthmatic children who are allergic to cockroaches are three times more likely to be hospitalised for their asthma if they live in a home with a large cockroach population.

Cockroach allergen is a protein found both on the insect's body (so a dead cockroach can still cause a reaction) and in its droppings. The allergens can become airborne with normal house dust, then inhaled. Because cockroaches contaminate food with their excrement, allergen can also be ingested at mealtimes.

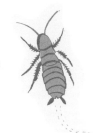

POLLEN

For one in six people in the United Kingdom and 35 million Americans, pollen is an extremely potent allergen. The condition that results from contact with these microscopic spores is a type of allergic rhinitis commonly known as hayfever. Pollen is carried by the wind, and during the spring and summer when pollen counts are high, large doses of this allergen are breathed in through the nose. When it comes into contact with the eyes and the sensitive, moist lining of the nose and sinuses, it sets off the allergic response in sensitive individuals. Hayfever sufferers usually react to at least one of the following airborne allergens: grass pollens from rye grass, timothy grass and other similar grasses; tree pollens from oak, elm, ash, birch or hazel; certain mould spores.

LATEX ALLERGY

Natural rubber latex is obtained by 'tapping' the rubber tree (*Hevea brasiliensis*), which grows in Africa and Asia. People who suspect an allergy to latex often experience their symptoms after wearing rubber gloves. They may in fact be reacting to chemicals such as household cleaning products, or their symptoms may be a result of incomplete hand-drying, repeated hand-washing, and sweating inside rubber gloves. True allergies to latex involve either a reaction to latex protein or to the chemicals added to raw rubber latex during harvesting, processing and manufacturing.

Sensitisation occurs after repeated contact with products containing latex, so it is generally regarded as an occupational hazard; for example, health-care workers are put at considerable risk through their daily contact with the material in the form of blood bags, gloves and other essential equipment. Children with latex allergy are likely to develop this condition because of an illness, such as spina bifida, which requires repeated surgical treatment and the use of catheters. Infants may develop an allergy after repeated contact with bottle teats and dummies.

Some people with a latex allergy also react to some common foods, including avocados, bananas, chestnuts, nectarines, papaya and peaches.

INSECT STING ALLERGY

Insects that are most likely to trigger an allergic reaction with their stings are members of the Hymenoptera family. This includes bees, wasps, hornets and fire ants. Allergic reactions are usually short-lived, lasting only a few hours, with redness and swelling followed by pain and itching. However, in some people reactions may last longer, and occasionally result in a life-threatening anaphylactic attack.

JEWELLERY (NICKEL) ALLERGY

Nickel is a malleable metal that is frequently used in metal alloys. Skin reactions to this potent allergen can be severe: people may be left with welts on their legs from the studs on their jeans, severe rashes on their wrists from nickel watch straps and blistered hands from touching nickel-rich cutlery. Nickel is found in most metal utensils in the kitchen as well as in costume jewellery, scissors, spectacle frames, buckles, zips, fasteners and coins. Some foods are also rich in nickel and can trigger a reaction when eaten by a few allergy sufferers. Foods high in nickel include: asparagus, cabbage, beans, corn, mushrooms, peas, tomatoes, spinach, sprouts, peanuts, pears, raisins, rhubarb, tea, herrings, oysters, baking powder, cocoa, wholemeal flour, all canned foods and all foods prepared with nickel utensils.

Indoor air quality

The air we breathe indoors is often laced with a cocktail of toxic substances. Indeed, the weight of scientific evidence suggests that indoor pollution has a greater impact on our health than outdoor pollution. In an average home, pollutants are so plentiful and diffuse that it can be difficult to identify the precise cause of a sufferer's ill-health.

ENDOCRINE-DISRUPTING CHEMICALS

Endocrine-disrupting chemicals are found in pesticides, PVC, preservatives, dioxin and lead, and experts suspect that it sometimes takes only a single exposure to these chemicals to disrupt normal cell functions. So little is known about endocrine-disrupting chemicals that safe exposure levels cannot be set.

Links have been established between the use of these chemicals and a range of serious health problems, from damage to the brain development of children, to the increased levels of breast, prostate and testicular cancer. Researchers in the United States are suggesting that girls are entering puberty earlier because of the chemicals to which their mothers were exposed during pregnancy.

The main culprits are building materials, paints, varnishes, technical equipment, cleaning products, furniture polish, air fresheners, combustion products from gas stoves, pesticides, synthetic fabrics, all kinds of smoke, and ambient air quality, including pollution from outside.

Toxic substances are made naturally by plants and animals to ward off predators and parasites, so it would be misleading to interpret the term 'natural' as meaning safe or non-toxic. But the fact remains that we are far more likely to be exposed to man-made toxins in our homes than to anything produced by the earth. Petrochemicals – derived from crude oil, a non-renewable resource – are the most diffuse synthetic substances. These substances are used in nearly every industry and every type of consumer product, despite the fact that many are known to release a range of chemicals and heavy metals into the air.

There is compelling evidence that domestic pollutants are triggers for allergies such as asthma. A multitude of common symptoms, including headaches and insomnia, are also linked to exposure to these toxins. Lastly, daily exposure to substances that mimic natural hormones is being implicated, at least partly, in the growing incidence of cancer, reduced fertility and birth defects.

One of the biggest problems is that no one knows exactly how harmful most indoor pollutants are, because the vast majority have not been fully tested. According to an estimate by the European Commission's Chemicals Bureau, only 14 per cent of the most widely used household chemicals have a full set of minimum safety data.

Whether or not a particular substance creates a toxic or allergic effect in an individual depends on a number of factors: the quantity to which that person is exposed; the strength of the substance; the method of exposure (some substances are safe to inhale but not to rub on the skin); the frequency of exposure; and an individual's tolerance.

However, even if your immune system is currently able to cope with a barrage of toxic substances, it would be presumptuous to assume that it will always be so robust.

There is no getting away from the fact that most indoor toxins are universally harmful to healthy people, and that the long-term effects of many substances are not known. Being aware of the risks makes it easier to minimise them.

A room-by-room inventory of the materials used to decorate and furnish a home will give you an idea of the chemicals in your living space. Foam-based sofas, synthetic fabrics, moth-proofed carpets and gloss paint all add to the toxic overload.

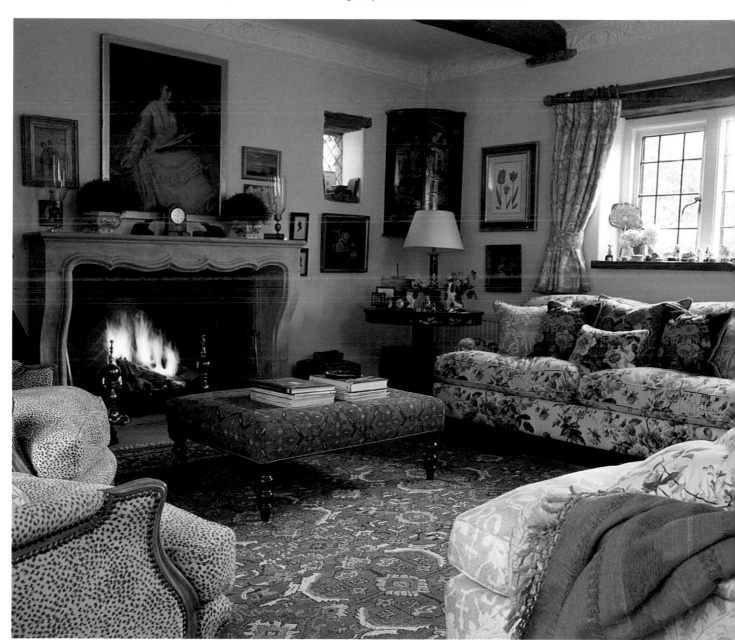

COMBUSTION POLLUTION

There was a time when indoor pollution meant one thing only: smoke. Soot found on the ceilings of prehistoric caves provides ample evidence that our forebears enjoyed the pleasures of an open wood fire. Five thousand years later, we tend to burn different materials in our homes and the pollution problems we face are less obvious. Clouds of black smoke have largely given way to the colourless and often odourless fumes produced by natural gas, fuel oil, and kerosene. Contributing to this whirling fusion of combustion by-products are space heaters, gas ovens, furnaces, gas boilers, gas clothes dryers, wood- or coal-burning stoves and fireplaces. Even a tiny, unvented gas pilot light produces undesirable fumes (mainly nitrogen dioxide). Adding to the load are exhausts from cars and lawn mowers, and fumes from hobby activities such as welding, woodturning and soldering.

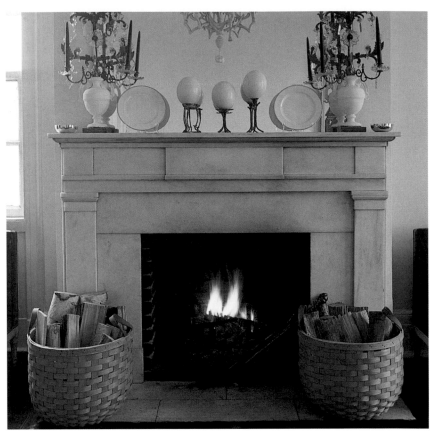

Most people have a vague awareness of these fumes and gases, but few waste time worrying about them – after all, these pollutants usually result from activities everyone depends upon, such as cooking and heating the home. But they have the potential to cause illnesses, allergies, disability, disease and even death in extreme cases. To make matters worse, combustion always produces water vapour, and though this is not usually considered a pollutant in itself, it can result in high humidity and wet surfaces, which encourage the growth of biological pollutants such as dust mites and mould.

If you live in a home that has an inadequate supply of fresh air or unvented, malfunctioning or improperly installed appliances, the following combustion gases may be compromising your health.

CARBON DIOXIDE

Carbon dioxide is the main combustion product from gas, kerosene, wood or coal. When appliances that run on any of these are in operation, concentrations of carbon dioxide in the ambient air rise significantly. It acts as a respiratory irritant and triggers feelings of stuffiness and discomfort.

CARBON MONOXIDE

This odourless, toxic gas is produced by the incomplete combustion of fuel. The symptoms resulting from chronic low-level exposure include headaches, fatigue, dizziness and nausea. Chronic exposure has been linked to Multiple Chemical Sensitivities (see page 18), as carbon monoxide can interfere with the detoxification pathways in the liver, causing toxic overload. Acute carbon monoxide poisoning is typically caused by faulty combustion appliances or those with malfunctioning external vents, and is the cause of around 60 deaths a year in England and Wales.

NITROGEN DIOXIDE

Exposure to nitrogen dioxide is thought to increase respiratory infections and coughing, particularly among vulnerable individuals such as children and asthmatics. In the home, nitrogen dioxide is produced by gas appliances, kerosene heaters and wood-burning stoves.

SULPHUR DIOXIDE

Sulphur dioxide is a colourless gas with a strong pungent odour. Long-term exposure has been linked to elevated asthma, breathlessness and wheezing. Concentrations are higher indoors than outdoors when kerosene heaters or poorly vented gas appliances and coal furnaces are used.

RESPIRABLE PARTICLES

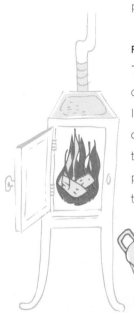

The smoke from burning fossil fuels results in the spread of 'respirable particles' in the air. These aerosols enter the lungs and lodge there, sometimes leading to airway constriction and a reduction in lung function. Woodsmoke, too, is believed to be associated with respiratory illness, particularly among vulnerable groups such as infants and those with pre-existing chronic respiratory disease.

Respirable particles became a dwindling problem when societies moved away from coal and wood-based fuels. However, now wood-burning stoves are back in fashion, the health problems associated with them are also making a comeback.

ENVIRONMENTAL TOBACCO SMOKE (ETS)

ETS is a mixture of the smoke given off by the burning end of a cigarette, pipe or cigar and the smoke exhaled from the lungs of smokers. The most common acute health effects are eye, nose and throat irritations. There is also a strong link between exposure to ETS and ear infections and acute childhood lower respiratory tract illnesses, such as bronchitis and pneumonia. A single smoker in the home doubles a baby's risk of developing asthma later in life.

RESPIRATORY IRRITANTS

Irritants do not in themselves trigger an allergic reaction, but aggravate the inflammation in a person's airway. Irritants make the symptoms of an allergy worse or more likely to occur. Examples of common irritants are cigarette smoke, petrol, paint and car exhaust fumes.

LEFT There's nothing more romantic or cosy than a real fire but, unless flues and vents are well maintained, toxic combustion by-products will build up inside the home.

BELOW Passive smoking is particularly harmful to people with allergies. However, even if you are allergy-free, smoke can make your eyes water as much as severe hayfever.

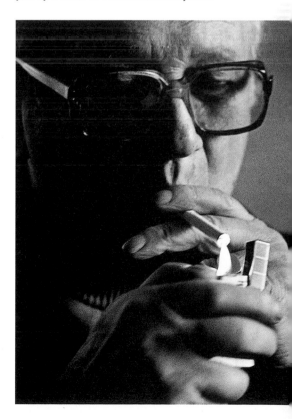

Building and decorating materials

Not so long ago, homes were put together using a much simpler range of materials than they are today. Wood, brick or stone formed the skeleton; the interior involved plastered walls, wooden floors and walls painted with simple paint formulations. Rooms were decorated with solid wood, and soft-furnishings composed of natural fibres such as cotton, wool, jute and silk. Synthetic components were rare, and building-related health hazards could be counted on one hand.

LEAD

The use of lead for roof flashing has increased over recent years. It is also used in synthetic dyes and PVC. Lead piping for water supply systems is still common in many countries and a source of drinking water contamination.

Lead used to be included in many paints to extend the durability of the coat. Then, these paints were found to be powerful neurotoxins, over-exposure to which can lead to brain damage. As a result, paint formulae were revised and paint containing more than 0.06 per cent lead by weight was banned. Today, lead is included in only a few specialist trade paints. However, millions of homes still contain contaminated walls and window frames and, when the paint peels or flakes, exposure levels can soon reach dangerous levels. Lead-painted sash windows can be problematic because, as they are raised and lowered over the years, paint erodes and dust may settle on window sills.

CADMIUM

This metal is a known kidney toxin and carcinogen, and is found in many PVC (vinyl or polyvinylchloride) materials, including vinyl flooring and window frames. Synthetic pigments made from petrochemicals (in particular red, orange and yellow) may contain cadmium.

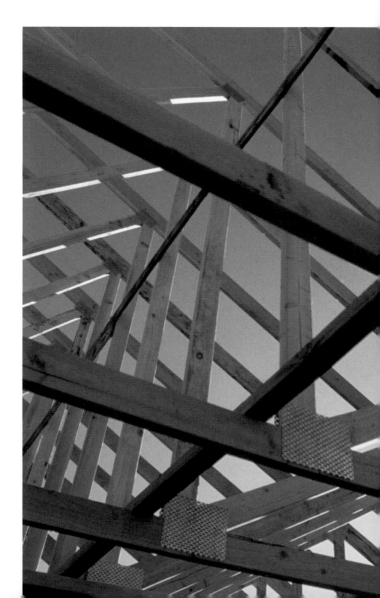

MERCURY

Mercury was formerly used as a fungicide in interior and exterior paints, and in drywall joint compounds. This highly toxic metal is still present in some water pipes, old paint-work, the backs of mirrors, and thermometers.

ARSENIC

This is used as a wood preservative, and can result in serious poisoning when wet wood is handled, though the greatest danger of contamination passes a few weeks after the wood has been treated.

VOLATILE ORGANIC COMPOUNDS (VOCS)

VOCs form the largest group of indoor air pollutants. They are derived from petrochemicals and are readily released as vapours in a process known as 'outgassing'. Some VOCs are air pollutants in their own right, but they also cause chemical reactions in the atmosphere that lead to the formation of smoge containing secondary pollutants, such as ground-level ozone. Asthmatics and people with other respiratory complaints appear particularly susceptible to low-dose VOC exposures, with nocturnal breathlessness reported as one of the main symptoms.

Because VOCs have good insulating properties, are fire-resistant and are cheap to produce, they have many applications in modern construction. They are an integral part of the solvents, resins and preservatives used to make composite wood products (such as chipboard, MDF and plywood), insulation products, carpets, glues, paints, and synthetic fabrics. The distinctive smell of 'new house' is caused primarily by such chemicals outgassing. VOCs are also found in household cleaning products, waxes, polishes, perfumes, synthetic soaps, and cosmetics.

Studies at Britain's Building Research Establishment have identified 254 VOCs emitted from building materials in the first year of the life of four newly built homes, and 71 during the second year. Two VOCs stand out from the pack and these are the ones discussed here: formaldehyde and benzene.

OUTGASSING

'Outgassing' describes the release of volatile organic compounds or VOCs from common building materials, furniture and other synthetic composites. Elevated temperatures generally increase the rate of outgassing.

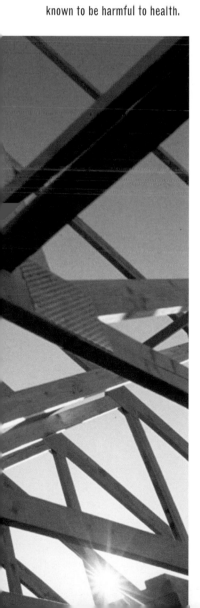

Solid wood has been phased out of building frames in recent decades and replaced with synthetic materials that are known to be harmful to health.

FORMALDEHYDE

Exposure to this colourless gas is starting to be recognised as a severe health hazard. Inhalation of formaldehyde vapour is thought to cause skin irritations, swelling and irritation of the throat, breathing difficulties, coughing, a burning sensation in the nasal passage, watery eyes, excessive thirst, tiredness, insomnia, headaches and disorientation. Exposure can also aggravate asthma attacks, and contact with formaldehyde finishes can result in skin rashes and exacerbate eczema. People who develop permanent health problems as a result of formaldehyde exposure often relate the onset of their symptoms to a flu-like illness, which is usually misdiagnosed as a viral infection. Because formaldehyde is an immune-system sensitiser, it may cause multiple allergies and sensitivities to entirely unrelated substances if exposure is chronic.

In the context of building materials, the largest sources of formaldehyde are composite wood materials, especially when these have not been given an impermeable surface.

This VOC is also used in the manufacture of urea formaldehyde foam insulation, and though its use is in decline because of health concerns, it is still injected into some wall cavities.

BENZENE

This is a known human carcinogen that is found in paints. Both conventional oil- and water-based paints contain VOCs, but it is the oil-based varieties that are considered more dangerous. A study of mortality rates among painters and decorators in Britain showed significantly elevated deaths from cancer compared to the rest of the population, a situation that has been attributed to benzene.

PAINTS AND FINISHES

People with allergies suffer in particular when exposed to the fumes in paint thinners and from those released as paint dries. Asthma flare-ups and skin irritations are common reactions to these toxins.

When decorating a room, colour and style are the most important elements. Few of us give much thought to the chemicals in our chosen materials.

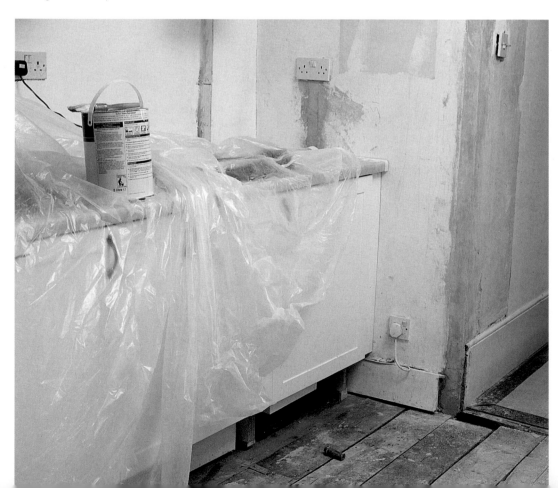

All paint is made from a combination of ingredients from four categories: resins, for adhesion and durability; pigments, which provide the colour; additives, which enhance performance properties; and solvents. A solvent is the liquid medium that allows paint and other products to penetrate porous materials. Concentrations are highest in products sold as 'solvent-based'; however, solvents are also found to a lesser extent in many water-based paints. Solvents evaporate as VOCs, causing health problems and serious pollution. They can trigger allergic reactions and damage the nervous system, the respiratory system, digestive organs, the circulatory system and the heart. They have also been linked to cancer and reproductive disorders.

Paints are classified according to the type of solvent they contain: oil-based paints contain 40 to 80 per cent VOC solvent, while water-based paints generally contain 5 to 10 per cent VOC solvent.

DO-IT-YOURSELF

Many home improvement projects are carried out under safety conditions that would not be tolerated in an industrial setting. A reaction may stem from large quantities of dust whipped up by tools, or it may be a reaction to the toxic fumes and vapours released from the materials being handled. This can trigger a new allergy or cause the flare-up of an existing one, in particular asthma, rhinitis or contact dermatitis.

PAINT STRIPPERS

Paint strippers contain methylene chloride, a very toxic chemical that has been linked to kidney disease, heart attacks and cancer. Methylene chloride is also a known source of carbon monoxide: the chemical is metabolised within the body to form this highly toxic gas. Even in a well-ventilated room, anyone using paint stripper will receive a hefty dose of methylene chloride.

ADHESIVES

Adhesives contain many of the same chemicals as paints and pose similar health risks. Skin complaints are the most common adverse reactions following exposure to toxic glues, from acute allergic reactions to longer-term dermatitis. Solvent-based adhesives present the greatest health hazards. Water-based products are safer to handle, though they often contain some solvents.

NEUROTOXINS

These chemicals are so called because they are toxic to the nervous system, which in turn affects every system in the body. Many neurotoxic substances are the same chemicals that cause cancer and Multiple Chemical Sensitivity (see page 18).

CARPETS

A cross-section of the average carpet reveals layer after layer of potentially hazardous material, from synthetic carpet fibres and backing to the synthetic underlay and solvent-based glues that sandwich together the various layers. A carpet may contain over 120 chemicals!

Americans first made an issue of floor coverings in 1988, when a new carpet was installed in the Washington headquarters of the Environmental Protection Agency and more than 10 per cent of the staff complained of health problems. Reported symptoms included burning eyes, memory loss, chills and fever, sore throat, joint pain, chest tightness, coughs, nausea, dizziness, blurred vision, depression and difficulty concentrating. It is widely believed that the culprit was the chemical 4-PC (4-phenyl-cyclohexene) released from the carpet's backing material.

One redeeming feature of new carpets is that their outgassing is at its peak in the first few days (though a few chemicals persist for up to three years). However, once in place, a carpet acts like a sponge. Biological allergens are the most obvious pollutants that sink into the fibres, but they are not alone: anything carried onto a carpet on shoes, such as VOCs, pesticides, and toxic household chemicals, can be stored then released back into the air. Away from ultraviolet sunlight, these chemicals can remain intact for many years.

SYNTHETIC FIBRES, BACKING AND UNDERLAY

Dozens of chemicals are released from the artificial fabrics used in cheap carpeting, but formaldehyde and benzene are usually cited as the greatest offenders. When a large area of flooring is being covered and ventilation is poor, the risks of becoming overexposed to these VOCs can be considerable. Synthetic latex (commonly used as a backing) also contains vulcanisation agents that include styrene, a carcinogenic chemical.

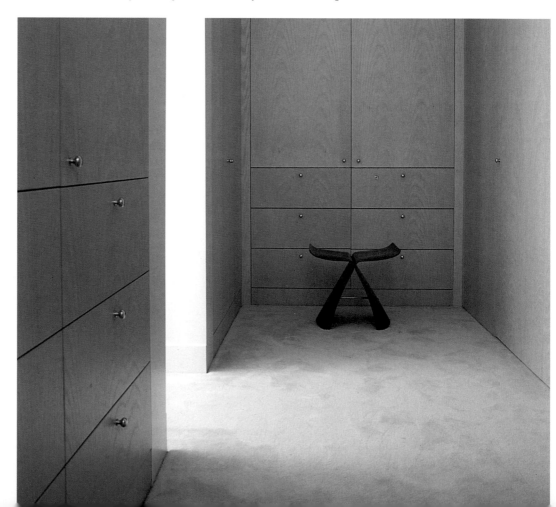

For softness and comfort, nothing beats carpet. But is a little luxury underfoot worth the price of a home laden with toxic chemicals? Choose natural, untreated carpets wherever possible.

POLYVINYLCHLORIDE

Polyvinylchloride (PVC) is the most common plastic used in the building industry, but its application is plagued by controversy for two reasons: its production and disposal are extremely damaging to the environment (it does not biodegrade), and its use indoors presents a range of alarming health hazards. It is thought that phthalates, a group of chemicals often added to vinyl, may contribute to indoor asthma incidences. The environmental group Greenpeace is campaigning for a worldwide end to all industrial chlorine chemistry, including the production of vinyl in all its forms.

Its common household usages include easy-wipe wallpaper and blinds, flooring, carpet backing, shower curtains and window frames.

ADHESIVES AND SEALANTS

Many types of glue are used in carpet installations, but the majority are based on synthetic latex, the same resin used in carpet backing. Although there are a growing number of 'safe' adhesives available, most installers still use glues that contain volatile solvents. These adhesives often provide the greatest short-term source of VOC emissions in the home.

CARPET TREATMENTS

Chemicals to inhibit stains, static and fungal growth have become standard in recent years, yet all of these treatments are potentially toxic. Another process that has a history of both health and environmental problems is the moth-proofing of wool carpets. (See 'Pesticides', page 60.) The synthetic dyes used to colour carpets also contain potentially harmful solvents and VOCs.

FABRICS

Fabrics that are not 100 per cent natural can cause problems for people with Multiple Chemical Sensitivities, those with a sensitivity to synthetic dyes or anyone with an intolerance to formaldehyde.

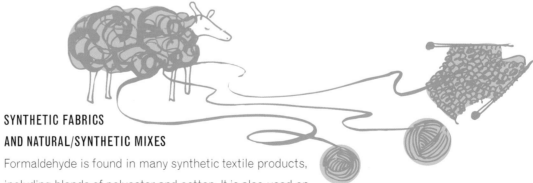

SYNTHETIC FABRICS AND NATURAL/SYNTHETIC MIXES

Formaldehyde is found in many synthetic textile products, including blends of polyester and cotton. It is also used on nylon fabrics to make them flameproof. Fabrics treated with formaldehyde resins are often described on their labels as 'crease resistant', 'easy care', 'no-iron', or 'water repellant'. Polyester and polycotton sheets are known to exacerbate eczema symptoms, probably because they 'breathe' less than cotton and linen and so lead to more sweating and skin irritation.

WOOL ALLERGY

Wool fibres are a very common irritant, especially among people with eczema or dermatitis. However, a few individuals are reacting to the lanolin in wool rather than the wool itself. Others may be sensitive to the bleaches, fungicides and synthetic dyes used in the treatment of their garment and may be fine wearing woollen clothes that have been coloured with natural pigments and have undergone no treatments.

Chemicals in your home

Around 100,000 different chemicals were in use in the European Union in 1981, the vast majority of which had not been adequately tested for toxicity. Since then, several thousand more have been added to the market. In 1998 a survey looked at every one of the 2,863 high-volume organic chemicals in use in the United States and concluded that a full set of basic toxicity information was available for only 7 per cent of these chemicals.

PESTICIDES

Anything that exterminates insects, rodents, weeds, fungi, bacteria or mildew is classified as a pesticide. House dust is an effective reservoir for older pesticides and a major source of human contamination – especially for infants and toddlers. The Environmental Protection Agency has found 23 pesticides in indoor dust and air.

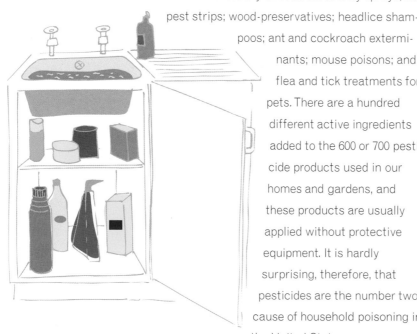

Pesticides usually exist as aerosol fly sprays; no-pest strips; wood-preservatives; headlice shampoos; ant and cockroach exterminants; mouse poisons; and flea and tick treatments for pets. There are a hundred different active ingredients added to the 600 or 700 pesticide products used in our homes and gardens, and these products are usually applied without protective equipment. It is hardly surprising, therefore, that pesticides are the number two cause of household poisoning in the United States.

Pesticides are stored in fatty tissue and can accumulate over time to dangerously high levels. When fat is burned during exercise or lost on a diet, (continued page 62)

OZONE

Ozone molecules play a vital role in the upper atmosphere, absorbing dangerous ultraviolet radiation from the sun. On Earth, ozone is a highly reactive oxygen compound that can irritate the lungs. Blurred vision and loss of concentration may also accompany these symptoms. In addition, ozone may worsen chronic respiratory diseases, such as asthma, and compromise the ability of the body to fight respiratory infections.

Electrical equipment such as brush-type motors (the type found in kitchen appliances, sewing machines and power tools), electronic air cleaners, negative-ion generators and photocopiers are the main sources of ozone in the home.

Ozone generators are marketed as air-purifying devices, but the concentration of ozone in the air needed to eliminate mould, insecticides, odours and toxic VOCs would have to be higher than humans can tolerate without risking their health.

COMMON HOUSEHOLD CHEMICALS

Chemicals act as allergy triggers in one of two ways: either the pollutant itself causes a direct effect by toxic damage (for example, on the lungs or on the skin), or exposure leads to sensitisation, making individuals susceptible to an allergic response upon contact with other indoor allergens. What follows is a list of chemicals and chemical groups that are causing particular alarm among environmental and health groups. They are all either toxic, persistent, bio-accumulative (i.e. they build up inside our bodies), hormonally disruptive, or a combination of the above.

ALKYLPHENOLPOLYETHOXYLATES AND RELATED SUBSTANCES

Used as surfactants, dispersants, and emulsifiers in some shampoos, shaving foams and other cosmetics. Also used as additives in some paints and epoxies, such as epoxy resin glue. These are endocrine-disrupting chemicals.

ALKYLTIN

Used as a preservative in antibacterial agents. Also used as catalysts in the production of some plastics. These compounds are persistent, bio-accumulative, endocrine disrupters.

ARSENIC

See page 55.

ARTIFICIAL MUSK SCENTS

Found in toilet cleaners, shaving foam, aftershaves, liquid soaps, cosmetics and perfumes. Not to be mistaken for natural musk extracted from the endangered musk deer, artificial musks accumulate in the body, contaminating fat, blood and breast milk. Synthetic musk is hard to avoid, as it is typically identified on a product label simply as 'perfume' or 'fragrance'.

BISPHENOL A

Used in the production of plastic bottles, epoxy glues, fire retardants, and the protective coatings inside some tin cans. Bisphenol A is an endocrine disrupter with a range of toxic effects.

CADMIUM

See page 54.

CHLORINE

Not only is chlorine bleach extremely dangerous if accidentally ingested, it also produces very harmful fumes. These cause skin irritations, headaches, fatigue, burning eyes and breathing difficulties. Chlorine is a very toxic and reactive chemical that combines with organic matter to form organochlorines. These compounds accumulate in our bodies and have been linked to birth defects, cancer and reproductive and developmental disorders.

DIOXINS

Produced as by-products in the manufacture of some other chemicals, for example PVC. Dioxins are persistent, bio-accumulative endocrine disrupters. The most researched dioxin, TCDD, is proven to cause cancer.

LEAD

See page 54.

MERCURY

See page 55.

PHTHALATES

These toxins are often present in household dust, and have been linked to incidences of asthma. Foetuses are known to absorb them through the placenta, and babies through their mothers' milk. Some phthalates are endocrine disrupters that have been linked to a reduction in sperm count, disruption in reproductive cycles and increased breast cancer rates.

SHORT-CHAINED CHLORINATED PARAFFINS (SCCPS)

Found in paints, mastics, sealants and fire retardants. Medium- and long-chain chlorinated paraffins are just as hazardous and should also be avoided. These are used in PVC cables and vinyl flooring. Short-chained chlorinated paraffins are suspected endocrine disrupters. They are persistent, toxic and bio-accumulative.

LINDANE

Lindane is a possible human carcinogen and has been linked with breast cancer, disruption of the endocrine system, aplastic anaemia and birth defects. It is banned in the European Union as an agricultural and gardening treatment; however, it is still used in a few domestic products including some ant and weevil killers, moth proofers and lice and scabies treatments. In the United States, the Environmental Protection Agency has classified lindane as a persistent, bio-accumulative, toxic chemical.

pesticides are released into the bloodstream. Within our bodies they attack the nervous system and trigger respiratory problems. The effects of pesticide exposure vary, depending on an individual's vulnerability at the time of exposure, the patterns of use and a person's genetic make-up. Some people have no reaction at first but develop extreme sensitivity to a product over time. Other people's bodies mount an immediate response.

Acute symptoms following pesticide exposure can often be mistaken for flu or an allergy. They include asthma-like reactions, skin irritations, nausea, dizziness, headaches, aching joints and muscles, sweating, disorientation, fatigue, inability to concentrate, hyper-excitability, moodiness, vomiting and convulsions. Scientists have also established links between chronic pesticide exposure and serious, long-term disease, including cancer, birth defects, genetic damage, decreased fertility, and sexual dysfunction. Pesticides are also supremely damaging to wildlife and highly polluting to the environment.

DUST MITE CONTROL

Chemical treatments, or 'acaricides', tend to be marketed as the best way to get rid of dust mite allergens. However, individuals with a dust mite allergy are the very people most susceptible to allergic reactions to such chemicals. Treatments are typically applied to carpets, upholstery, and bedding: places where young children spend most of their time. The British-based Pesticide Action Network UK believes this leads to undesirable exposure to pesticides over a long period of time and is unnecessary when non-chemical solutions exist. Research compiled by them shows that, in the short term, these treatments can lead to eye and skin irritations, while long-term complications include endocrine disruption, skin sensitisation and foetal toxicity.

Sixty years ago, virtually no preservative treatments were carried out on timber; today public exposure to toxic wood treatments is widespread and uncontrolled throughout the developed world.

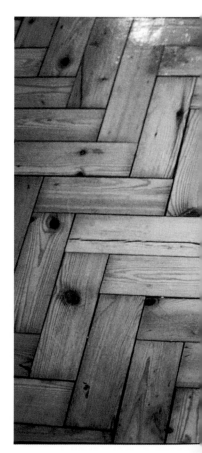

COMMON PESTICIDES

The families of domestic pesticides that are causing most alarm are organophosphates, pyrethroids, and carbamates, along with the active ingredient fipronil. In the United States, chlorpyrifos is the most widely used insecticide: it is known to be highly toxic to wildlife and has been linked to Multiple Chemical Sensitivity. A 1998 study found that chlorpyrifos accumulated in furniture, toys and other absorbant surfaces up to two weeks after application.

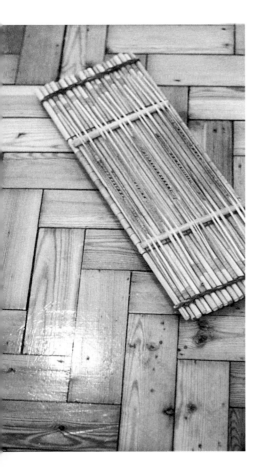

INSECT REPELLANTS

The most commonly used chemical in insect repellants is DEET (common name for diethyl-metal-toluamide). DEET has been linked with brain disorders, slurred speech, difficulty walking, tremors, acute neurotoxicity in children if accidentally swallowed and sometimes death. Until fairly recently, the United States allowed products with less than 15 per cent DEET to be applied on children, but in April 1998 America's Environmental Protection Agency stated that it could no longer certify that DEET was 'safe' for children.

MOTHBALLS

Traditional mothballs are made from 100 per cent paradichlorobenzene, which smells vile and is linked to a number of unpleasant symptoms after prolonged exposure. These include swollen eyes, severe irritation to the nose, throat and lungs, headaches, loss of appetite, depression and liver and kidney injury. Just one ball swallowed by a young child will result in seizures within the hour.

TIMBER TREATMENTS

Wood preservatives – used to exterminate wood-boring insects and fungus – are among the most toxic chemicals known. The long-term effects of exposure are unknown, yet public exposure to wood preservatives is widespread and uncontrolled. In the United States, timber treatments represent over 30 per cent of all pesticide use.

In the United Kingdom, an estimated 200,000 wood treatments are undertaken in homes each year, with an estimated 4 million dwellings (one-fifth of the total housing stock) having been treated during the past 25 years. To compound the situation, around a quarter of properties receive multi-treatments.

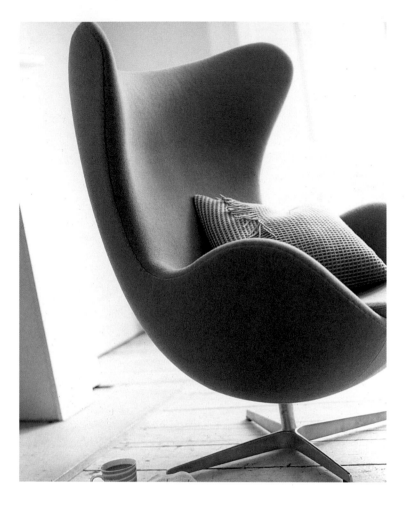

Much modern furniture is treated with flame retardants in order to protect our welfare. But toxic residues have been detected in human blood and breast milk. They have also been found in the air in offices that have treated electronic equipment.

CHRONIC HEALTH EFFECT

'Chronic health effect' refers to an illness that is a result of repeated exposures to a chemical over a long period of time. The contaminant can be hard to identify and the symptoms may not show up for years. The result of chronic exposure can be the onset of a new allergy; a chronic illness such as cancer; fertility problems or sexual dysfunction.

FLAME RETARDANTS

Desirable though it may be to protect people from injury and death from fire, the fumes released during the production, use and disposal of materials treated with flame retardant chemicals are alarmingly toxic. They are suspected carcinogens and have been linked to liver tumours and disruption of the endocrine system. In 1998, the World Health Organisation recommended that brominated flame retardants be phased out altogether.

Flame retardants are mainly used to treat the flexible polyurethane foam used in furniture and upholstery, and the casings, covers, circuit boards and other components of computers. New, less hazardous materials are commercially available that are intrinsically flame-resistant, and manufacturers of electrical and electronic equipment are starting to reconsider their options. A number of well-known companies are moving away from using brominated flame retardants in their products. Among these are the computer manufacturer Toshiba and furniture superstore IKEA. Sony has made a commitment to phase out brominated flame retardants in its products by 2002. Flame retardants have been replaced in the housing of most television sets manufactured since 1997.

CLEANING PRODUCTS

Cleaning products are among the most toxic substances kept in the average home. But though there is growing suspicion that some of these products may be implicated in cancer, liver damage, lung problems, suppressed immune systems and damage to foetuses, there is nothing on the labels that hints at long-term effects. Furthermore, products sold in aerosol containers are known to exacerbate existing allergic conditions, especially asthma, and both the British Allergy Foundation and the American Lung Association warn against the use of aerosol sprays.

Hazardous substances are found in most commercial brands of household products, including general-purpose cleaners, dish-washing products, drain cleaners, oven cleaners, dishwashing powders, window-washing liquids and furniture waxes and polishes. Chemicals used in dry-cleaning present further problems, and even laundry detergent can trigger reactions in some people: the residues can cause severe rashes, and the artificial fragrances that linger in the air can lead to flu- and asthma-like symptoms.

WATER

Our supposedly fresh water supply never delivers pure H_2O. Sediment is a common contaminant, but more worrisome are the nitrates, chlorine, pesticides, aluminium and other heavy metals (including lead, copper, cadmium and mercury), organic matter and industrial chemical residues that seep into the water system. These pollutants can make unfiltered water an irritant for people with allergies, chemical sensitivities and skin disorders, whether it is ingested or used on the skin. Of particular concern (especially to young children and people with eczema) are chlorine and fluoride. A true allergy to chlorine is uncommon, but anyone whose eczema is made worse by swimming in a chlorinated pool may be affected by chlorine in their home's water supply.

Fluoride is added to water supplies to reduce dental cavities in children, but too much fluoride can weaken the immune system and cause heart disease, genetic damage and cancer. Children who drink treated tap water and use flouride toothpaste may be exceeding a safe level of intake. Consult your local water company if your are concerned.

MEDICINE

Non-prescription drugs are formulated to relieve symptoms, not to cure the underlying problem, so they should be taken with caution. What is more, some drugs are known allergens and others have side effects that are nearly as unpleasant as the problems they set out to mask. Allergy sufferers should be wary of non-prescription medicine: it is easy to fall into a pill-popping routine to smother symptoms while the underlying condition persists or even deteriorates, unnoticed and unchecked.

As many as one person in three experiences some form of adverse reaction to a drug, though this is often drowsiness, nausea or a headache rather than an allergic response. Nevertheless, true allergies to drugs do arise. Indeed, the most common cause of anaphylactic shock is an allergy to commonly used medicines, ointments, creams, sprays, serums in vaccines, local anaesthetics, and desensitising injections for allergies.

Allergic reactions to drugs can be slow or immediate, trivial or life-threatening. Previous exposure to a drug is required for a sensitivity to surface, though the initial exposure may have occurred just one day before in cases where a course of drugs is taken continuously over a number of days. Sometimes a drug is tolerated for weeks, months or years before sensitisation develops. The allergic reaction may be to the drug itself or to other components of the medication, such as dyes, bulk fillers, preservatives, antibacterial substances and colourings.

The medicines most likely to trigger a reaction are aspirin (two out of every thousand people are allergic to aspirin), anti-inflammatory painkillers such as ibuprofen, the antibiotic penicillin and beta-blocker drugs used to treat high blood pressure.

BEAUTY PRODUCTS

It is a surprising fact that laws in the European Union do not require that cosmetics be tested for safety before they go on sale. Many manufacturers like to boast that their ingredients are 'natural' and 'kind', yet in the next breath they point to the years of cutting-edge research that have gone into their latest creations. If a cosmetic contains even one synthetic ingredient (and the vast majority contain many), it has no rightful claim to the tag 'natural'. But what most consumers do not realise is that dozens of the ingredients routinely added to hair and beauty products are either allergenic, hazardous, or of unproven toxicity. These preservatives, additives, and chemicals are intended to make the preparations smell nice and feel smooth and luxurious on the hair or skin. They are also there to stop the product from breaking down too fast, going mouldy, or harbouring bacteria. Particularly toxic and hazardous are many of the ingredients added to hair products, especially those formulated to dye, wave or straighten tresses.

Rashes and contact dermatitis are the most common reactions to hair and beauty products, but allergic reactions can also occur after exposure to airborne vapours,

COSMETIC CHEMICALS

The following chemicals are known to cause allergies or allergy-like symptoms.

ALCOHOL

Often the active ingredient in commercial astringents and toners, it is also used in many cleansers. Can cause allergic reactions and dry skin; fumes can irritate nasal passages and cause nausea, drowsiness and dizziness.

FORMALDEHYDE

Found in some shampoos and all nail hardeners. Formaldehyde is a potent VOC known to trigger allergies and create chemical sensitivities. (See also page 56.)

ISOTHIOZOLINONE

Used widely in cosmetics, isothiozolinone is a common allergen linked to contact dermatitis. People have been known to react to tiny amounts. (Isothiozolinone is a pesticide derived from synthetic pyrethroid permethrin and is also used as an anti-dust-mite agent.)

LAUREL SULPHATES

Found in most commercial bar soaps, liquid detergents, shampoos, and creamy cleansers. These are synthetic detergents made from petroleum or an extracted plant fatty acid. Considered harmful to human skin and mucous membranes, and widely believed to cause skin rashes and allergic reactions, these substances may also form carcinogenic compounds when mixed with certain other chemicals.

PARABENS

Methyl-, ethyl-, propyl- and butyl-paraben are used to extend the life of cosmetic and food products and to inhibit microbial growth. Thought to cause allergic reactions and rashes.

PROPYLENE GLYCOL

Used as a solvent, propylene glycol renders preparations less thick than they would be if made from glycerol. It also inhibits the growth of mould and is sometimes used for its moderate bactericidal qualities. In spray solutions, it can be used to stabilise the size of droplets. This chemical is a known skin and respiratory irritant. Over-exposure is thought to cause liver abnormalities and kidney damage.

SODIUM HYDROXIDE

Used in nail treatments and as a hair straightener. If it comes in contact with the eyes, sodium hydroxide can cause blindness.

THIOGLYCOLATE

Mixed into hair-straighteners and wave lotions, thioglycolate is a serious eye irritant and is known to cause skin sensitisation.

droplets and particles of various cosmetics. And the human skin is an organ with strong powers of absorption, so chemicals are easily drawn into the body. Beauty products that most commonly trigger allergies are face and body creams, sunscreens, deodorants, shaving products, aftershave and hair care products. It is worth noting that the most expensive products are not necessarily the best.

SOAP AND OTHER SKIN CLEANSING PRODUCTS

Many of the soap-like bars sold in the shops are not soaps at all, but cakes of synthesised chemicals containing petroleum-based detergents. These are often highly drying and irritating to sensitive skin. Even commercial bars that legitimately call themselves soap are rarely made in the basic way of reacting natural oils and fats with an alkali. Instead, they are usually made from chemically extracted fatty acids reacted under high pressure with alkali.

BUBBLEBATHS

Commercial preparations are usually made from a synthetic detergent with added artificial fragrance and a generous dash of man-made dye. Using bubblebath can lead to skin rashes and infections of the urinary tract, bladder, kidneys and vagina.

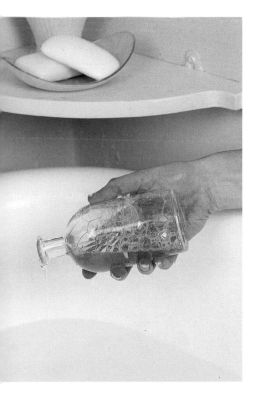

ABOVE Filling your bath tub with a luxurious head of foam may seem like harmless indulgence, but shop-bought bubblebath is entirely artificial and can cause skin rashes.

RIGHT Commercial soaps may look enticing, but they often contain a raft of unsavoury products. Check labels before you buy.

BABY PRODUCTS

Mainstream brands usually contain mineral oil (a petrochemical), synthetic detergents, artificial fragrances and preservatives. They are often harsh on a baby's delicate skin and can lead to allergic rashes.

SUNCARE PRODUCTS

The ingredients that are most likely to produce an allergic response are cinnamates (octyl methoxcinnamate and cinoxate), benzophenones and PABA (now dropped from most products because it caused a range of reactions). The preservatives and alcohol in suncare products can be further sources of irritation.

FRAGRANCE

Reactions to fragrances range from mild skin irritation to severe rashes and contact allergy. Migraines and nausea are other effects.

Perfume consists of a combination of natural essential oils, flavours, chemicals and solvents in a base of alcohol. Any one cosmetic product may contain as few as ten or as many as 600 ingredients. Dermatologists have identified just 24 fragrance ingredients as common allergens, but these are present in most products.

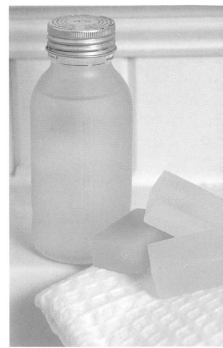

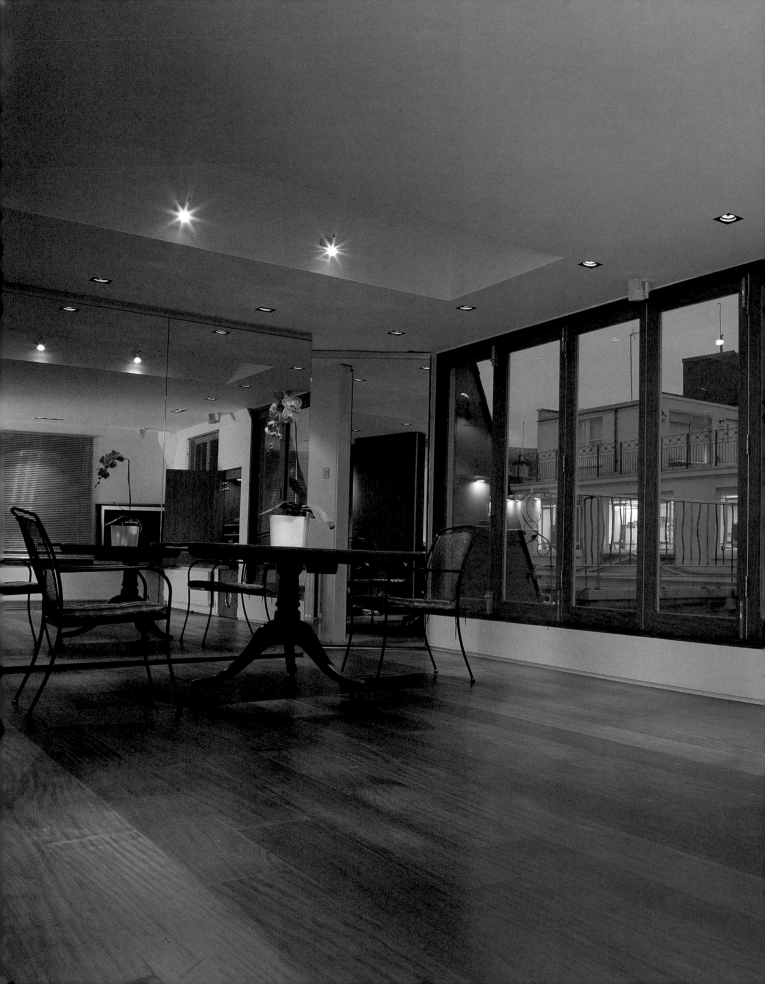

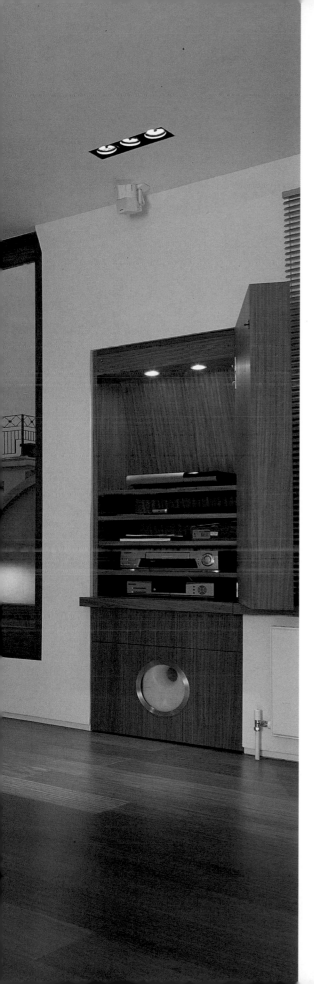

solutions

Few of us lie awake at night worrying about house-hold pollution, and the mention of indoor allergens does not send waves of panic through the population. Though both allergens and domestic pollution pose a powerful threat to health, they are invisible forces with low public profiles and are easily overlooked as topics of concern. But the evidence, once it has been laid out before you, is nearly impossible to ignore. Suddenly you become aware that your home is swarming with potentially harmful life forms; that your kitchen is a soup of hazardous gases; that the chemicals stashed under your sink are untested poisons; that the expensive perfume you dab behind your ears is a powerful allergen; and that even the wood of your bookshelves may be poisoning you. In short, you learn that there is probably nothing Alpine fresh about your indoor environment, no matter how sweetly you have scented it with air freshener.

HEALTHY HOME FATIGUE

It is hardly surprising that some people, once all the contributing risk factors have been considered, succumb to 'Healthy Home Fatigue', the philosophy of which goes something like this: 'There is so much in my home that is wrong, I don't know where to start putting things right, and in any case I probably can't afford to see the project through, so I think I'll bury my head in the sand instead'.

In some ways this rationale cannot be faulted: an overhaul of your home is expensive and complex. But before throwing in the towel, you should consider this: most people can make considerable improvements to their home's bill of health by making a few straightforward changes that will not leave them bankrupt. Once these improvements have been made, rather than fretting over past decisions, aim to make wise ongoing decisions in the way you run, update and (occasionally) overhaul your household. That is where this book aims to help.

Do not allow yourself to become intimidated by the huge scope for change in your home. Remember, there is no prescribed order in which to make improvements; every reader should first focus on the specific issues affecting his or her health and then address future concerns. The directory of allergy services, mail-order companies and useful products listed in the Sources section (see page 120) is designed to help turn battle plans into direct action.

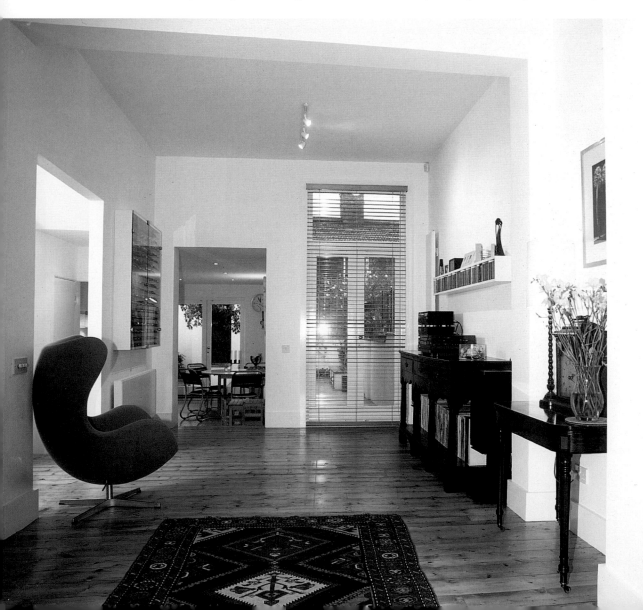

Although there is no need to panic, there are three strong arguments for taking your offensive one step further and waging war against all common allergens and indoor pollutants:

1 Allergy sufferers are likely to develop other allergies over time, so reduction of exposure to known allergens should be of long term benefit. This is particularly true of the house-dust mite: researchers have no doubt that there is a relationship between an individual's level of exposure to mite allergens and the risk of becoming sensitised to mites, which could lead to asthma later in life.

2 Environmental pollutants and irritants make many pre-existing allergic conditions worse because they aggravate any existing inflammation of body tissue.

3 Babies who are exposed to allergens and other environmental pollutants early are more likely to develop an allergic disease later in life.

Take heart from the knowledge that many measures aimed at reducing one type of allergen load also reduce levels of others. However, when it comes to decontaminating your home, patience pays. The hyper-irritable state that can be created by allergens in your home may take several weeks after the last exposure to settle completely, so the benefits of control measures take time to be appreciated.

LEFT AND RIGHT Once you've decided to make your home a healthier place, don't be put off by the magnitude of the task; a few simple steps can make all the difference. The changes you make don't need to cost the earth: wooden floors and washable furniture covers make excellent and often inexpensive alternatives to synthetics.

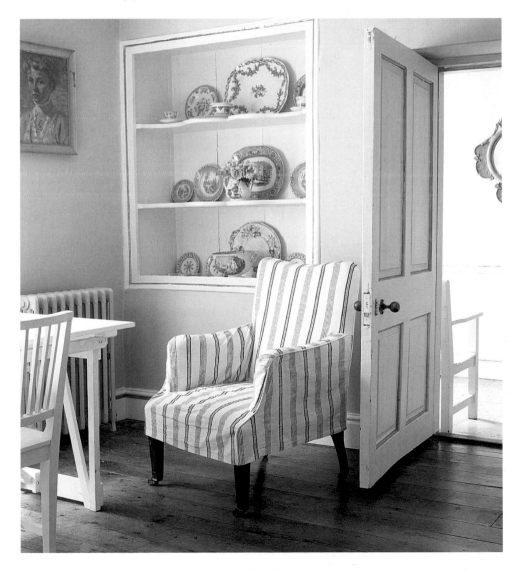

Avoiding common indoor allergens

The most compelling reason to reduce allergens and pollutants is also the most obvious one: these irritants are directly responsible for the allergies and ill-health suffered by you and/or other members of your household. Therefore, your long-term aim should be to stop all common allergens in their tracks and avoid new sources of indoor air pollution.

DUST MITES

Some visitors simply cannot be persuaded to leave a home no matter how unwelcome you make them feel, and dust mites are the most persistent of guests. In any given mite colony, there are simply too many fast-breeding individuals for total extermination to be feasible. And even if you were to achieve the amazing feat of tweezing the last of the mites from your mattress, a new colony would take up residence right away. So resign yourself: if the conditions in your home are warm and moist, mites will remain part of the fabric of your home. But you should not focus too obsessively on mites, as it is your exposure to their allergen that matters. Reducing mite numbers today will reduce your exposure to fresh allergen tonight, but it will have no effect on the allergen that has been accumulating for years. To reduce your exposure to fresh and old dust mite allergen, your campaign should be two-pronged: attack on fresh allergens and protection from existing allergens.

STRATEGIES FOR THE BEDROOM

Four simple steps can reduce dust mite allergen in the bedroom to 10 per cent of their original level. These are: ventilate the room well, keep humidity low, frequently clean carpets with a powerful vacuum cleaner, and use allergen-barrier covers.

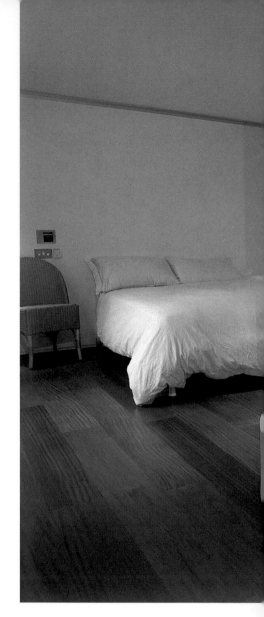

ABOVE Make dust mites feel unwelcome in your bedroom by minimising shelving, taking up carpets, and using sheets that can be washed at high temperatures.

ABOVE RIGHT Replacing curtains with wipeable blinds makes it even harder for mites to take up residence.

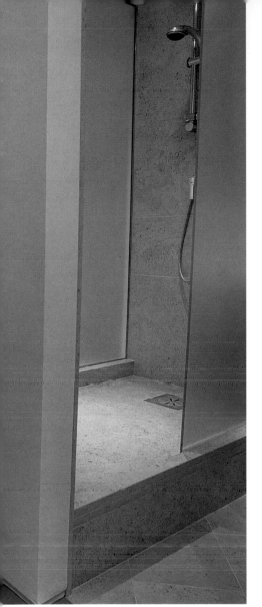

ATTACK ON FRESH ALLERGENS:

◆ Dust mite allergens dissolve in water of any temperature; however, the mites themselves are destroyed only in hot water, so bed linen should be put through a weekly wash at 55 to 60°C (130 to 140°F). Most cotton bed linen can withstand these temperatures. An alternative is to use chemicals called acaricides. (See page 76.)

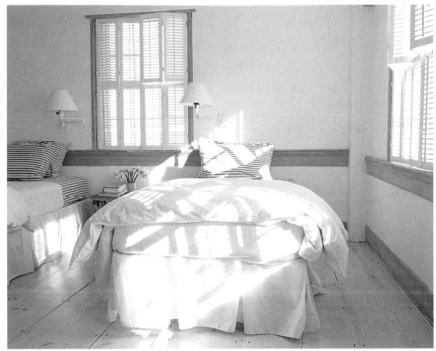

◆ Pillows, quilts, duvets and blankets that cannot be washed every week at high temperatures (such as those with fillings made of wool and feathers) should be replaced with synthetic or foam equivalents. These are both less conducive to mite growth and can withstand a hotter wash cycle.

◆ Use light, washable cotton curtains and wash them frequently.

◆ Where possible, remove carpeting. Carpets are an important habitat for dust mites, and the older the carpeting, the greater the concentration of allergens.

◆ Where carpet removal is impractical, vacuum often, as this helps remove dead mite bodies and faecal pellets that are light enough to become airborne when disturbed.

However, vacuuming does not remove live mites, which hang on to the fibres with suckers and hooks on their legs. Moreover, in the short term, vacuuming increases the concentration of airborne allergens, so it is best done in the morning. If you are asthmatic, use a mask and stay out of the room for at least 30 minutes afterwards.

◆ Store clothing in closed cupboards or drawers.

◆ On a sunny day, hang bedding outside to air. Dust mites will perish when exposed to two hours of ultraviolet light.

◆ Damp-dust all surfaces frequently.

◆ A final word on bedding: when shopping for new fabric, be cautious of the term hypoallergenic. This means the fibres themselves do not cause allergy; nevertheless, all fibres (especially natural ones) can harbour dust mites.

PROTECTION FROM EXISTING ALLERGENS:

◆ The best way to maintain a distance between yourself and the existing allergen in your bed is to enclose the mattress in an allergen-barrier cover that traps existing allergens and cuts mites off from their food source. Covers are sold in major department stores and by mail order. They can be bought fairly cheaply; however, at the bottom end of the market, covers are usually made of plastic and are uncomfortable to sleep on. More expensive versions are made of a polyester-cotton fabric and feel similar to normal sheets (though polyester is a man-made fibre and has its disadvantages). The best covers form a complete barrier to all particles, while allowing water vapour to escape. Check that the product has a minimum perme-ability index of 40 per cent according to British Standard 7209, and preferably greater than 75 per cent. (Barrier covers made from EPFTE are highly efficient.) Mattresses should be totally encased in the cover and closed with a zip, so avoid those that work like fitted sheets.

◆ Allergens will continue to accumulate on top of and inside allergen-barrier covers, so it is essential to damp wipe covers when you change the bed linen and allow them to dry thoroughly.

◆ If you are reluctant to replace delicate wool and feather pillows, quilts, duvets and blankets with synthetic fabrics, encase these, too, in allergen barriers.

◆ If you prefer to start your fight against dust mite allergen with a clean slate, you can call on the services of specialists who heat-treat household items. Mattresses, pillows, duvets and soft toys are enclosed in a massive envelope and heated to 100°C (212°F) for at least one hour, killing all mites and denaturing the allergen.

CHILDREN AND DUST MITES

Be careful with allergen-barrier covers: there is a risk of suffocation if a child puts his or her head inside. Keep covers zipped up when in use and out of the reach of children when not. Allergen-barrier mattress covers should not be used for babies under six months, but are safe after that age. The main allergy agencies do not advise the use of acari-cides in children's bedrooms (see page 76). Do not allow children to play on beds – this stirs up allergens.

Buy soft toys that are washable in hot water. If a toy does not fit this crite-rion, wash it once a month in cool water to remove the allergen, then place it in a plastic bag in the freezer for six to 12 hours to kill the mites. Repeat at least once a month. Incidentally, even toys marked 'surface-wash only' seem to survive a spin in the cold-cycle.

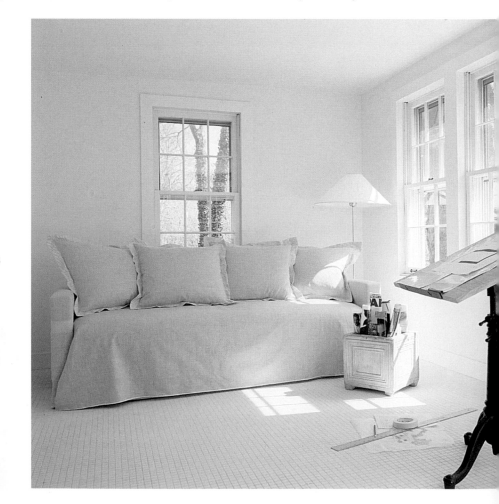

RIGHT By taking the minimalist approach, you will provide fewer surfaces on which dust – and dust mites – can settle.

LEFT Loose sofa covers can look extremely stylish in a modern living room. So long as they are washable at high temperatures, they can be regularly relieved of their dust mite colonies, too.

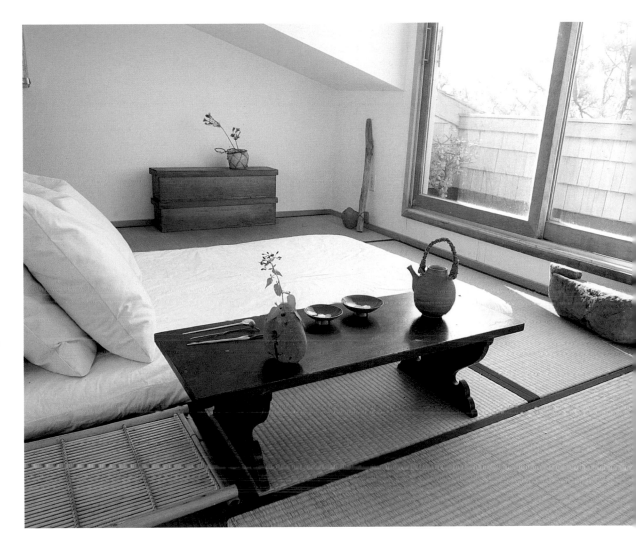

STRATEGIES FOR LIVING AREAS

Once you have addressed the problem of dust mite allergen in the bedroom, the fight should be broadened to include the rest of the home, starting in the living areas in which allergic individuals spend the most time.

SHORT-TERM MEASURES:

◆ Reduce the number of soft furnishings in each room. Also, dispose of knick-knacks or invest in display cabinets: all objects accumulate dust.

◆ Vacuum upholstered furniture regularly.

◆ Dust with a damp cloth.

◆ In hot homes, reduce the heat. Mites do not reproduce well below 25°C (77°F).

◆ Maintain low indoor humidity: keep kitchen and bathroom doors closed when cooking or running hot water, and do not boil kettles and pans in poorly ventilated areas. Do not dry washing indoors. Humidity levels can be measured by hygrometers, which are available at hardware stores. Mites begin to die at 40 to 50 per cent relative humidity.

◆ Increase ventilation by opening windows, and do not block open chimneys. In 'tight' energy-efficient modern houses, it may be necessary to introduce some form of mechanical ventilation.

◆ Air soft furnishings in the sun to kill mites.

◆ As a last resort . . . carpets and soft furnishings can be chemically treated to kill dust mites or neutralise the allergen (see Acaricides page 76).

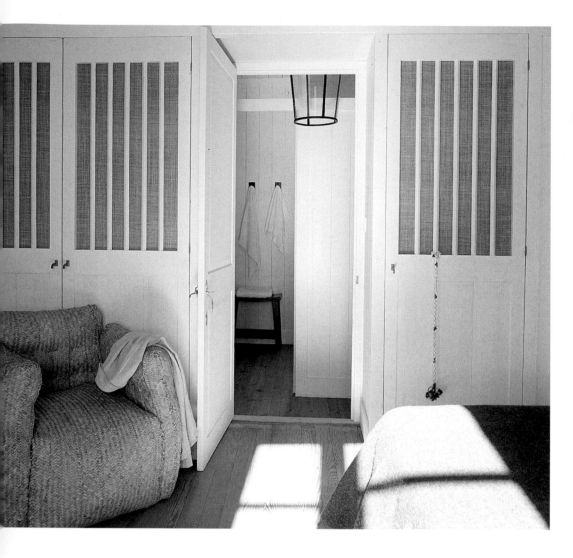

ACARICIDES

Acaricides are pesticides and some doctors have reservations about their long-term use. Their application on bedding, especially where children or pregnant women are likely to sleep, is not recommended.

Manufacturers of synthetic pyrethroids (bioallenthin, phenothrim, d-phenothrin, and isothiozolinone) claim these insecticides break down within a few hours of exposure to light. But light does not reach deep inside a carpet and potentially toxic levels could build up.

Tannic acid is the active ingredient in several commercial sprays and powders. This substance modifies dust mite and cat dander allergens, making them less likely to trigger reactions. However, these products don't kill mites and therefore require daily use to reduce the effects of the continual production of allergen.

As a final word: people tend to find it technically and financially difficult to treat complete houses with dust-mite killing chemicals.

ABOVE Worth exploring are the many alternatives to upholstered furniture. From rattan and wicker to bamboo and seagrass, these easy-clean, natural materials can be woven to look contemporary or traditional to please all tastes.

ABOVE RIGHT Rugs made from seagrass, jute and coir are easy to vacuum and provide a more inhospitable environment for dust mites than wool.

MEDIUM-TERM MEASURES:

◆ Replace carpets with hard floors.

◆ Dispose of upholstered sofas and chairs and replace with furniture that has removable covers that are washable in hot water, or cover upholstered furniture with allergen-barrier covers. Wherever possible, opt for leather furniture, as dust mites can be wiped off with a cloth.

◆ Replace heavy curtains and drapes with lightweight, washable cotton curtains or blinds.

◆ If the home's relative humidity is above 50 per cent, consider installing air conditioning.

◆ Ensure that air filters are kept clean on central heating systems and air conditioning equipment.

◆ Use dehumidifiers in damp basements.

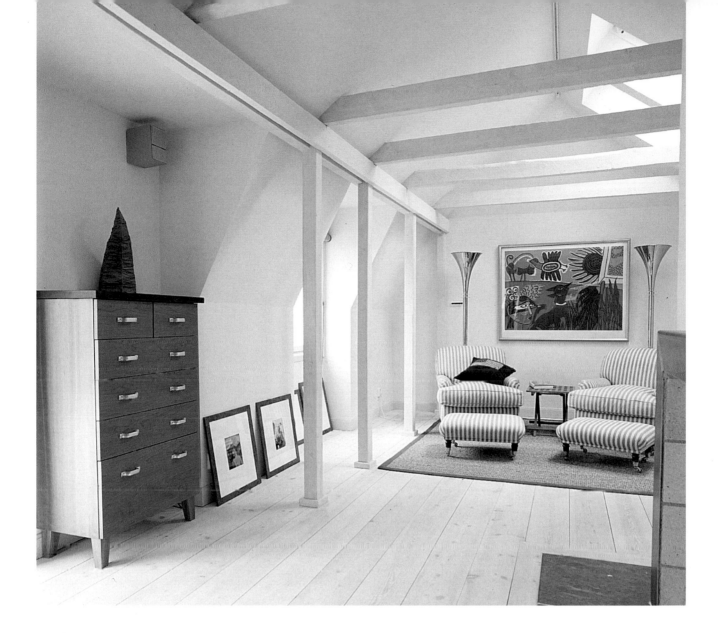

PETS

The problem with domestic animals is that people tend to fall in love with them and, even after discovering an allergy to a pet, most owners are understandably reluctant to boot them out. This being the case, the emphasis should be on reducing pet allergens throughout the house and eliminating them from sleeping areas. Reducing allergens can be achieved in the following ways:

◆ **Never** allow pets into the bedroom.

◆ Even if your pets never enter bedrooms, use the same precautions with bedding as described for dust mite control. Airborne allergens travel!

◆ Do not allow animals to make themselves comfortable in living areas.

◆ Open the windows often to aid ventilation and decrease airborne animal dander throughout the home.

◆ Ask a non-allergic person to groom dogs several times a week outside.

◆ Wash pet bedding every week.

◆ Ideally, shampoo cats and dogs twice weekly and treat them with a product that denatures allergens. (Get the pet used to being shampooed from an early age.) If this is unfeasible, buy a denaturing product that can be applied to the walls and furniture rather than to the pet's coat.

◆ If re-housing the pet is out of the question, at least do not buy a new one.

◆ If you are allergic to cat allergen and moving into a new home where you suspect a cat once lived, wash down the walls to remove residual allergen. Cat allergen can cling to walls even years after a cat has left and is easily stirred when someone brushes past. One study found that cat allergen can be reduced by 90 per cent when both pets and furniture are regularly washed. However, achieving this level can take many months.

MOULD, FUNGI, AND SPORES

Mould and fungi can grow on virtually any surface, but to take root and release their spores, they must find both a humid environment and a source of organic matter. Basement apartments, which are damp by nature, are easily the most problematic homes for individuals who form an allergy to spores. Here are some effective techniques for minimising their growth indoors:

◆ Maintain a well-ventilated, low-humidity home. Open windows for half an hour twice a day: this is an effective way to reduce indoor humidity and the growth of mould.

◆ In particularly damp rooms, invest in a dehumidifier.

◆ Open windows and close the doors to the kitchen and bathroom when running hot water or cooking.

◆ Do not pack clothes too tightly in wardrobes.

◆ Clean mould off refrigerators, windows and walls. Rinse and dry thoroughly.

◆ Remove fungal spores from contaminated objects.

◆ Regularly clean surfaces that are prone to mould, particularly in kitchens and bathrooms.

◆ Reduce house plants, as fungi grow in the soil. Change the soil regularly if you must have plants. (For the benefits of house plants, see page 97.)

◆ Regularly empty rubbish bins, as stagnant waste provides a perfect environment for mould.

◆ Wash bath mats frequently, as these are a common source of fungal contamination.

Keep bath rims mould-free by regularly repairing or changing the seal. To keep condensation in check, add moisture-absorbing plants to your bathroom. Boston fern and Kimberley Queen are particularly effective.

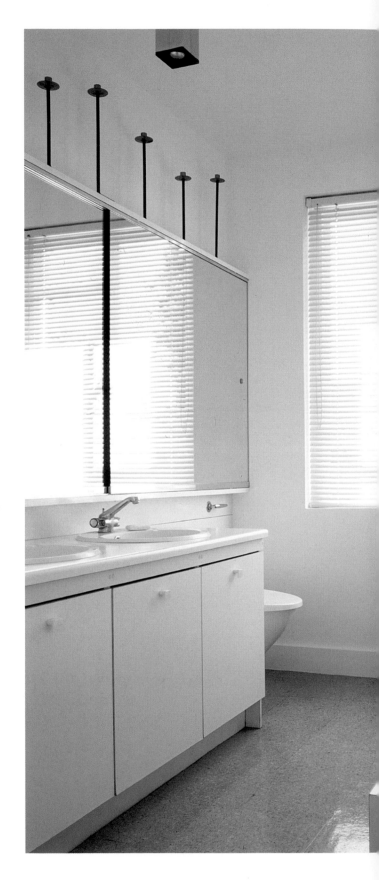

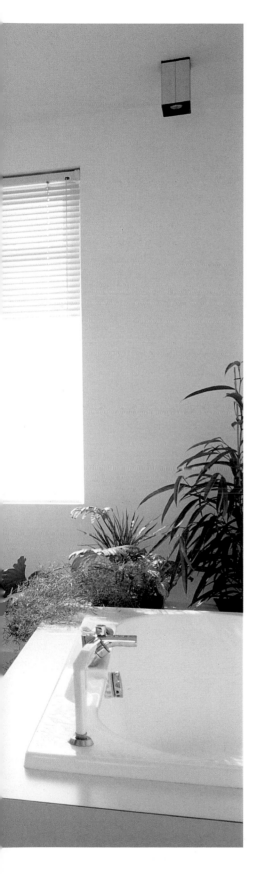

COCKROACHES

Cockroaches have not thrived on Earth for 400 million years by being wimps. They reproduce quickly, they duck and dodge many household pesticides, and after a seemingly successful extermination campaign they re-infest quickly by scuttling along drains and air ducts connecting one home to the next. It is said that they would survive nuclear fallout. So, we should concentrate our efforts on keeping the numbers passing through our homes to an acceptable level. The US National Coalition Against the Misuse of Pesticides recommends the occupants of every building set an 'action threshold' – that is, a level at which cockroach populations start to be considered unacceptable. Here are steps you can take to keep infestations well below this threshold:

◆ Store food in airtight containers.

◆ Clean up all food crumbs or spilled liquids immediately.

◆ At night, ensure that worktops and tables are wiped, sinks cleaned and floors swept. Cockroaches are most active after dark.

◆ Do not leave rubbish bins open.

◆ Keep cabinets clean and free from dust.

◆ Wash dishes as soon as they are used.

◆ Fix plumbing leaks and other moisture problems.

◆ In tropical climates, consider reducing the humidity with air conditioning or a dehumidifier.

◆ Do not store paper bags and cardboard boxes in the home as these make perfect homes and meals for cockroaches.

◆ Keep your home in good decorative order and free from excessive clutter: cockroaches eat carbohydrates as a first choice, but they also eat flaking paint, wallpaper pastes and book bindings.

If the infestation in your home is such that extermination is the only remedy, it is worth remembering that commercial products designed to kill cockroaches are toxic for people as well as pests. Here are some alternative pest-control measures you might like to try first:

◆ Set cucumber peel out on counter tops overnight to repel roaches.

◆ Fill a jam jar half-full with a mixture of beer, a few slices of banana or some other sweet fruit, and some drops of anise extract. Wrap masking tape around the outside of the jar to give cockroaches a foothold. Finally, smear a band of petroleum jelly around the inside rim to stop trapped cockroaches from climbing out.

◆ Give cockroaches a boozy send-off by soaking a rag in beer and placing it in a shallow dish overnight in an infested area. In the morning, send the drunken roaches to their grave.

◆ Sprinkle diatomaceous earth (pure silica) around floors, cracks and crevices.

◆ Mix borax with brown sugar and flour and sprinkle behind appliances and in corners. Cockroaches carry it back to their nests where it poisons the rest of the colony. (NB borax should be treated with caution – see page 101.)

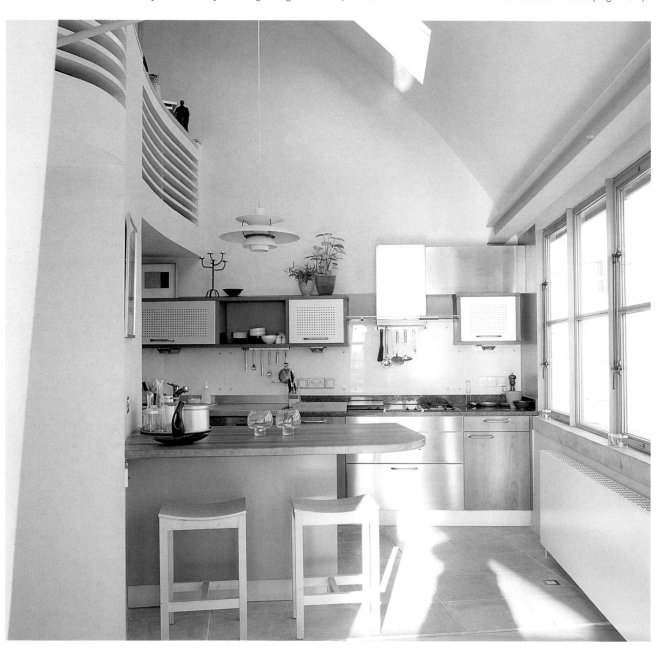

If you eventually feel compelled to resort to chemical pesticides, use the least toxic formulations you can find. Here are some pointers:

◆ Use poison baits or traps first before pesticidal sprays.

◆ Favour a formulation of 99 per cent boric acid. Boric acid is a naturally occurring mineral that is a very effective cockroach stomach poison. (Do bear in mind that as a poison it should be handled with care. Use only in areas where it will not come into contact with people or animals, such as in cracks and crevices and behind counters.)

◆ If you resort to sprays: limit them to the infested area; do not spray where you prepare or store food or where children play or sleep; do not spray when asthmatics are present; keep the window open while you spray; air the room thoroughly after spraying.

POLLEN

Pollen allergy is a common and often debilitating condition, but generally it becomes a problem indoors only when windows are left open during the day in the pollen season. If outdoor pollen counts are high:

◆ Remain indoors or at least limit outdoor trips. On warm, dry days avoid being outdoors during late morning and early evening when pollen counts usually peak.

◆ Keep windows closed when indoors or open them only after dark, when pollen levels are at their lowest.

◆ Keep windows in the car rolled up while driving.

◆ Avoid mowing lawns.

◆ Wear wraparound sunglasses.

◆ Change clothes and wash hair after spending time outside to remove trapped pollen.

◆ Take holidays by the sea, where pollen counts are usually lower.

LEFT Cockroaches love sticky work tops and unswept floors, so even if you're tidy in the kitchen, you may need to review your cleaning practices.

RIGHT Pollen-allergy sufferers often learn to live without cut flowers in their homes. However, it is possible to appreciate the fruits of spring without suffering unduly by asking your florist to trim the stamens from the centre of each flower when you buy them.

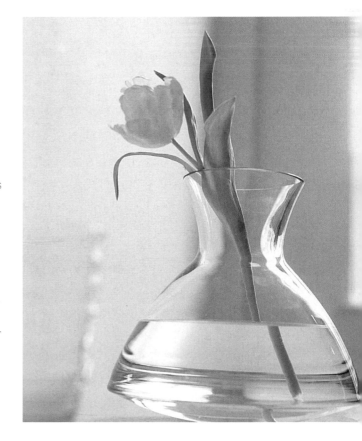

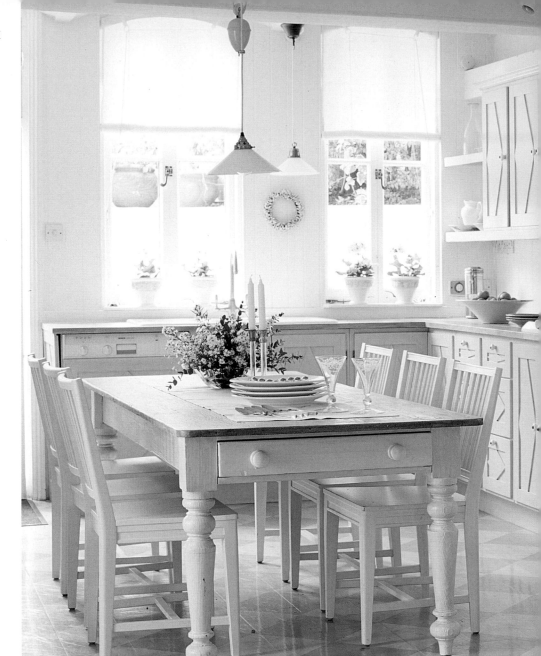

The kitchen can be a hazardous place for the allergic individual, but making cooking and eating places safer need not be complicated. Open windows more frequently and for longer, and opt for natural materials. You can't beat solid wood flooring brightened up with environmentally friendly paint.

LATEX ALLERGY

Reaction to natural rubber latex is not uncommon, yet this provocative material is used in thousands of everyday items, from pharmaceutical gloves to condoms, rubber boots, elastic bands, pencil erasers, the elastic in gloves and socks, sports equipment, car interiors and furniture. Non-latex gloves are now available and elastane (Lycra) is an obvious alternative to latex in clothing.

Allergic individuals are also advised to avoid the weeping fig (*Ficus benjamina*), as the presence of this common house plant is known to exacerbate symptoms.

As far as condoms are concerned, it is not usually the rubber proteins in latex to which individuals are allergic, but the preservatives and accelerators used in their manufacture. So in the first instance it may be worth simply switching condom brand. Some people overcome a true latex allergy by using a natural membrane condom under the latex condom if the allergy affects the male, or over the latex condom if it affects the female. Caution: a natural membrane alone does not provide adequate protection against sexually transmitted diseases. Polyurethane condoms are another option for allergic individuals.

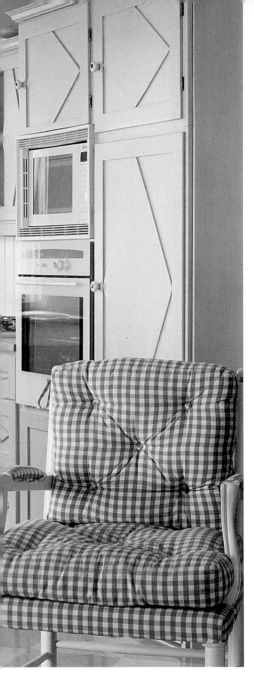

INSECT STING ALLERGY

Obviously, it is when you are outdoors that you are most at risk of encountering an insect with a sting in its tail. However, specimens do occasionally wing their way into the house, so it is advisable for allergic individuals to avoid going barefoot in summer, to wear closed-toe slippers, and to avoid standing under eaves of houses or near dustbins where insects tend to congregate. Keep an emergency treatment kit nearby at all times. Stings demand the following immediate treatment:

◆ When possible, remove the stinger and scrape over the area with a fingernail. Do not squeeze, as this may force venom into the body.

◆ If there is any risk of anaphylaxis, seek emergency care at once.

JEWELLERY (NICKEL) ALLERGY

If you are allergic to nickel, either eliminate objects containing this metal from your kitchen, wardrobe and jewellery box or create a barrier between the metal and your skin. Here are some tips:

◆ Use kitchen utensils, saucepans and scissors made from aluminium or stainless steel, and opt for implements with wooden or plastic handles.

◆ Wherever possible, buy clothes with non-metallic zips and other fasteners.

◆ Wear jewellery items with a higher gold content, or else wear platinum or stainless steel. It is often the earring 'butterfly' rather than the decorative front that triggers an allergic response, but surgical steel backings are a safe alternative and can be bought from most jewellers.

◆ Items such as watches and keys usually contain nickel, and if they cannot be avoided, they can at least be coated with several layers of clear nail polish, lacquer or a plastic coating that is sold by some jewellers.

◆ If you are severely allergic, avoid foods rich in nickel. However, if your condition does not improve, return to a normal diet. Most allergic people are not affected by foods with a high nickel content.

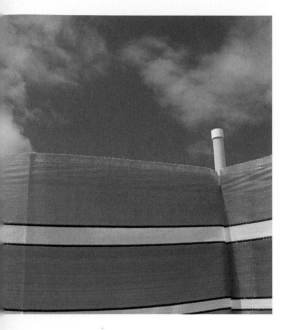

Improving indoor air quality

Air that is free from excessive contaminants is one of the best investments you can make for your long-term well-being. Because direct links have been made between many common household pollutants and allergies – particularly asthma and eczema – if you or any members of your household are affected by one of these conditions, it is doubly important to address the issue.

If you suspect something seriously wrong with the quality of the air in your home, you should have it analysed professionally. Contact the Environment Health Department for your area, who either will have their own testing facilities or will send you a list of analytical laboratories.

REDUCING COMBUSTION POLLUTION

Kitchens and utility rooms should have a health warning slapped on them for all the pollutant particles and harmful gases they spew into the rest of the house. Here are steps you can take to minimise the risks of overexposure:

GAS APPLIANCES

◆ Improperly installed appliances can release dangerous pollutants and may create a fire hazard. Be sure that the installer checks for back-drafting on all vented appliances.

◆ Ensure that all appliances are regularly serviced.

◆ When cooking, catch gases before they can contaminate the rest of the house by installing a high-quality extractor fan above your stove. (Carbon-filtered fan hoods re-circulate the majority of combustion pollutants back into the room.) Fit a duct, chimney or pipe to carry the combustion pollutants outside. In the absence of a vent, open a window during cooking as toxic gases accumulate

around the appliance then spread to the rest of the home.

◆ Ensure that ventilation and filtration systems are kept clean. If they fall into a state of neglect, these systems are likely to add to the concentrations of indoor pollutants by harbouring dangerous bacteria, fungal toxins and VOCs.

◆ Choose a gas stove with an electric igniter.

◆ Regularly check stove burners for blockages.

◆ If you are buying a new boiler choose a 'sealed combustion unit'.

◆ Ask a properly trained engineer (or CORGI-registered plumber in the United Kingdom) to service your central heating system once a year.

◆ Install a carbon monoxide detector device (available from hardware and DIY stores).

◆ Consider replacing some or all of your gas and oil appliances with electric units. This will reduce combustion by-products in your home.

WOOD-BURNING STOVES AND OPEN FIRES

◆ Choose an airtight wood-burning stove instead of an open stove or an open fire.

◆ Maintain good ventilation during operation: wherever possible, open windows as well as flues, fans and vents.

◆ Use seasoned hardwoods (elm, maple, oak) rather than

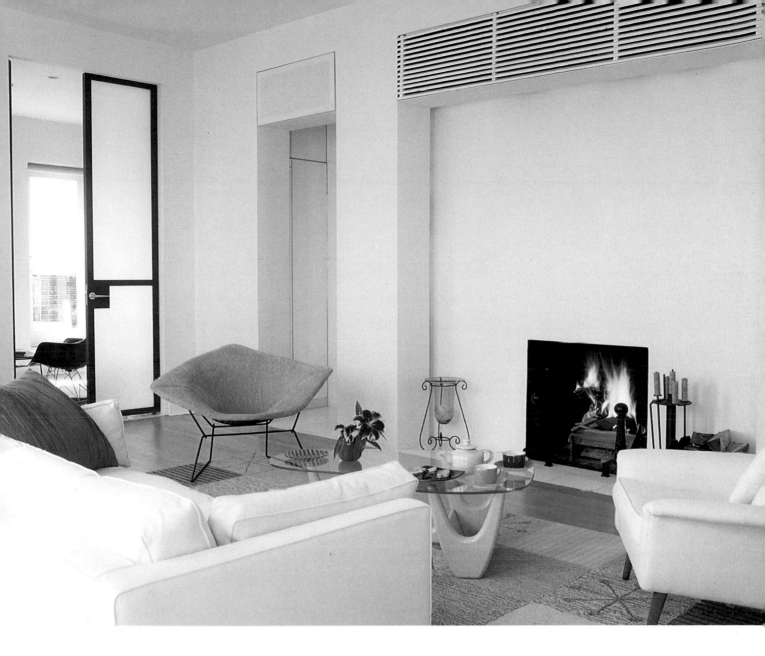

If you have a wood-burning stove, watch out for smoke, a layer of soot on furniture or a constant smoky smell; these are signs that the flue is not working properly.

softwoods (cedar, fir, pine). Never burn painted wood or wood treated with preservatives, because these could release highly toxic pollutants, such as arsenic or lead. Don't burn plastics, charcoal or coloured paper (including comics) as they too produce toxic gases.

GAS SPACE HEATERS AND KEROSENE HEATERS

◆ Always follow the warning labels and instructions.
◆ Buy appliances that are the correct size for the area to be heated. Using the wrong size heater could produce more pollutants and is not an efficient use of energy.
◆ Keep doors open to the room in which you are using an unvented heater and leave a window slightly ajar.

Building and decorating materials

The sources of pollution in most homes are multiple, and few are the people with the time or resources to rebuild interiors from scratch, ripping up carpets and replacing PVC window frames and particleboard furniture overnight. So where pollution is inevitable, keep windows open as much as the weather permits and consider purchasing an air filter. What follows is a review of other measures that will make your home more hospitable. Remember: a healthy home can be built one manageable step at a time!

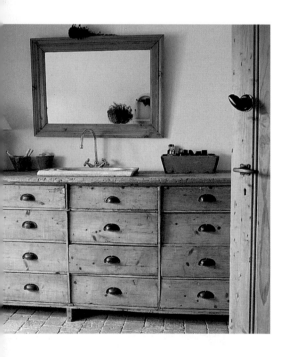

SOLID FURNITURE

Favour solid wood items over composite-bonded materials, such as particleboard, plywood or medium-density fibre-board (MDF). Although formaldehyde is a preservative found naturally in wood, it is the synthetic resin found in large quantities in composite wood products that gives rise to health concerns.

◆ Never cut composite-bonded materials inside the house, and wear a mask even when cutting them outside.

◆ Try one of the 'green' materials on the market. These include Tectan, a chipboard-like material made from used beverage cartons; Wheat-Straw Particleboard, made from chopped wheat straw mixed with a resin and pressed into panels; and Trex Lumber, an alternative decking material made from recycled plastic bags, industrial stretch film, sawdust from furniture factories, and wooden pallets.

◆ If you are obliged to keep items of furniture containing formaldehyde, seal in the fumes with a natural paint finish. A vapour barrier is most effective, though it will need to be reapplied every few years.

◆ Prevent formaldehyde fumes from building up inside wood veneer cabinets by lining them with heavy duty aluminium foil. Foil tape can be used to seal the edges.

LEFT AND RIGHT Solid wood is always preferable to MDF or particle-board. Leather sofas and chairs are immeasurably better than vinyl.

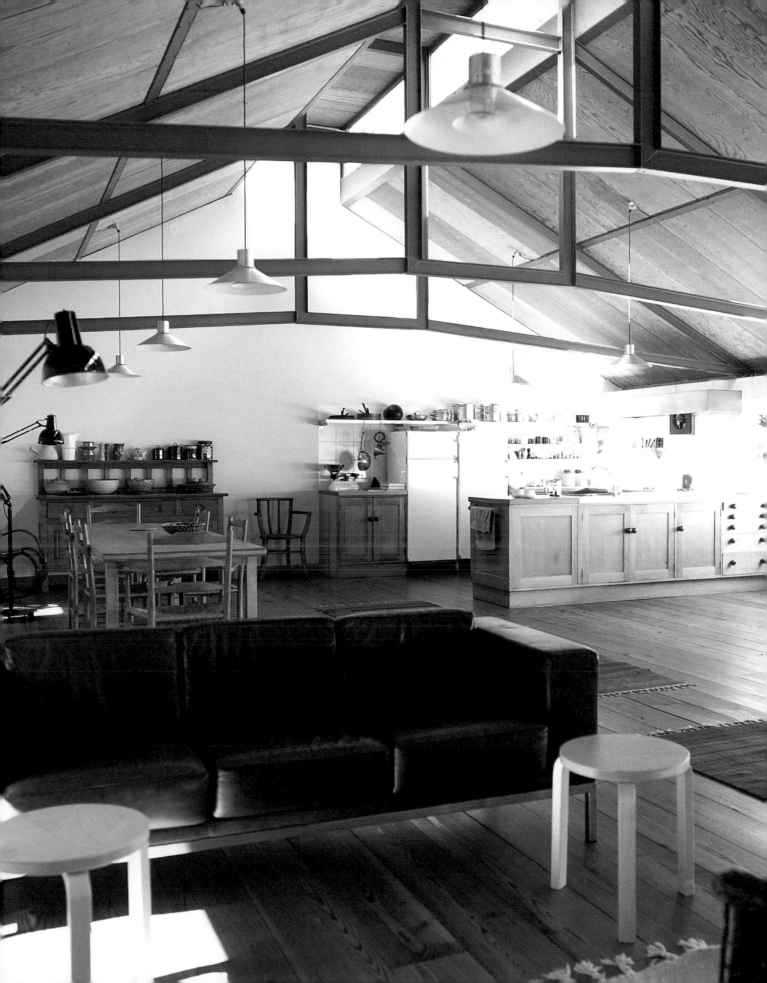

DO-IT-YOURSELF

Always protect your body and hands by wearing long-sleeved clothing and rubber gloves. Wear a well-fitting mask that has been designed to filter out specific airborne pollutants, such as dust, cement or fumes. Here are some other points to bear in mind:

◆ Favour water-based products over solvent-based ones.

◆ Choose products that contain natural raw materials or low-outgassing synthetic materials.

◆ Use a natural solvent (such as genuine balsamic turpentine oil or citrus peel oil) rather than a turpentine substitute or white spirit, both of which are petroleum-based. Note, however, that natural solvents are toxic and should be applied only in a well-ventilated environment.

◆ When using adhesives, caulking material, lubricants, glues, damp-proofing fluid or any other home maintenance material sold in a pot or a tube, maintain a well-ventilated work area and seal it off from the rest of the home.

◆ Choose water-based sealants that inhibit the outgassing of VOCs from composite wood products.

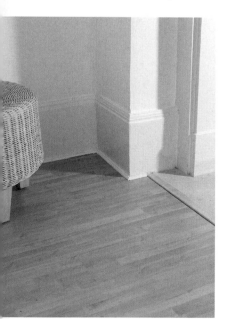

LEFT The manufacturers would have us believe that anyone can lay a laminate floor, but before throwing yourself into such a project, make sure you become an expert on adhesives and underlays.

RIGHT Hardwood floors can be expensive, but are the ideal choice for people who react to the dust mites that lurk in carpets and rugs.

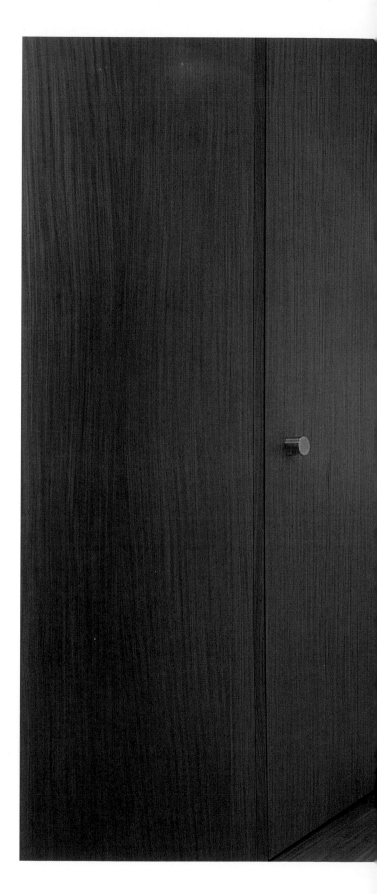

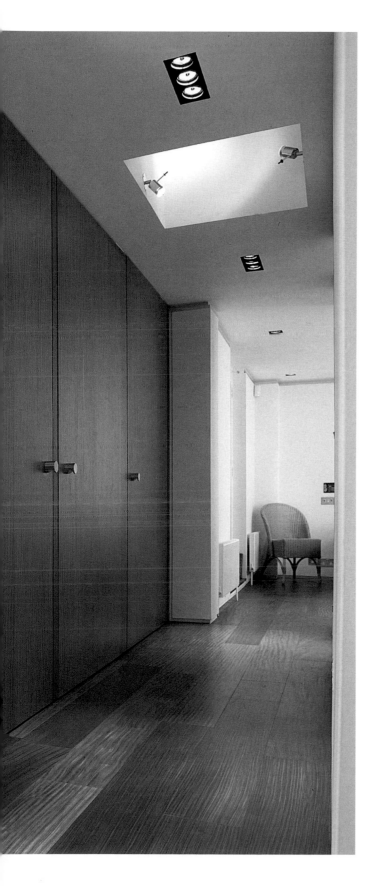

◆ Avoid solvent-based glues, such as epoxy resins, formaldehyde-based glues or acrylic glues. Consider using lower toxicity alternatives instead. Best of all, use a natural glue manufactured from soy, blood albumen or casein.

◆ Avoid urea-formaldehyde foam insulation. Choose flax, wool, recycled newspaper (in the form of loose fill cellulose and in batt form) or wood fibre board.

TIMBER TREATMENTS

Avoid the need to treat indoor wood altogether by good practice. The best way to overcome wood rot is to fix water leaks, provide good ventilation and dry out the air with air conditioning or central heating. Though dry rot travels across dry sections of timber, it needs a water source to flourish. If treatment is inevitable, keep the following points in mind:

◆ Avoid chemical wood treatments and, when buying new wood, check that it has not received a precautionary treatment, such as a fungicide to prevent rot or an insecticide to prevent woodworm attack.

◆ If chemical treatment is the only option, favour boron-based preservatives over all others. Next best are water-based zinc, copper, or fluoride compounds.

◆ In particular, avoid solvent-borne organic preservatives. Lindane, pentachlorophenol and tributyl tin oxide are especially toxic.

◆ After using any kind of chemical treatments, ventilate the relevant room well.

◆ When cutting or sanding wood – and especially chemically treated timber – wear a protective mask and vacuum the area thoroughly afterward to remove smaller particles.

◆ More often than not preservatives are needed only in high risk areas, such as windowsills, so opt for localised rather than blanket treatments.

◆ To prime wood, use oils and resins that living trees and plants produce to nourish and protect themselves from rot and insect attack. These substances penetrate the timber fibres, giving new timber deep protection and rejuvenating old, weathered wood.

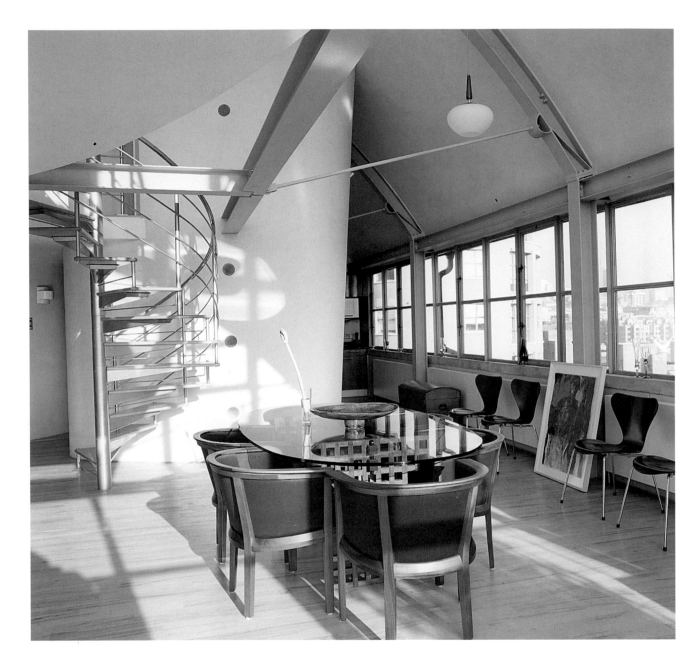

PAINTS AND FINISHES

For a healthy home, use paint that contains no or few VOC components and a low concentration of toxic chemicals. For a paint to receive the 'eco' label in European Union countries, it must contain roughly half current typical levels of VOCs. In the United States, the Green Seal Award is given to paints that have a low VOC content and do not contain toxic chemicals including benzene, toluene cadmium, and formaldehyde.

This is a good time to be shopping for natural plant-based paints, as there is a growing number of alternatives on the market. When these substitutes are used, outgassing is a much less serious problem, as VOC levels are extremely low (however, good ventilation is still essential). Also, painted surfaces are less conducive to static and attract less dust, which can be a significant bonus for allergy sufferers. The best natural paints are both water-proof and microporous, which means they allow moisture to pass through them so there is less blistering and flaking of paint. Here are some tips on buying and using green – or greener – paints and stains:

◆ Always choose water-based paints and stains.

◆ Be wary of solvent-based paints that are advertised as odourless. The main risk is when occupants ignore instructions to ventilate the room, or use the room too early after applying the paint, thus increasing their exposure to a strong concentration of solvent.

◆ Be cautious when using shellac. This is a thermoplastic resin material dissolved in alcohol, and is often used both as a clear paint finish and in paint effects. It is highly toxic both in skin contact and inhalation. However, shellac outgasses quickly and is usually safe in a matter of days.

PAINT STRIPPERS

◆ Avoid methylene chloride-based products and solvent-based strippers that use other toxic and flammable ingredients, such as toluene, methanol and acetone.

◆ Strippers that contain pine-oil/surfactant blends or phenol-based surfactants are safer and less flammable than traditional ones, but require more time to dissolve thick layers of paint.

◆ Do not start to strip paint or wallpaper if there is any chance that old layers of lead paint may lurk below. Also, regularly inspect windowsills and door frames where friction can grind down paint layers. If surfaces are intact, do not disturb them. If you suspect a problem, contact your Environment Health Department, who will give you advice on removing the contaminated paint.

◆ If using a blow torch, protect yourself from toxic gases by wearing an organic vapour mask, seal off the area to be treated and keep it well ventilated. When sanding or scraping old paint layers, wear a mask and vacuum up the residual dust.

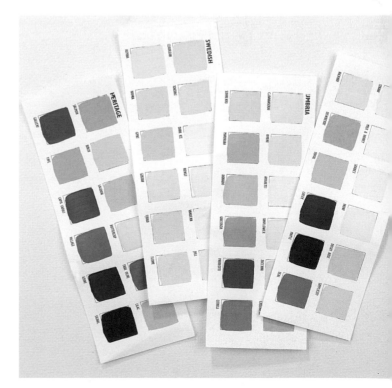

LEFT Wherever possible, buy paints that have a low VOC content (these are invariably the more expensive option). Better still, avoid synthetic paints and stains altogether and opt for a plant-based alternative. Nowadays, these come in a wide range of alluring colours such as the ones shown below.

CARPETS

The United Kingdom has the highest use of carpets in the world – 98 per cent of British homes are thought to have wall-to-wall carpeting – and 70 per cent of floors in the United States are covered by carpets and rugs. By contrast, just 2 per cent of homes in Italy are carpeted.

If you count yourself among those who simply would not live without soft pile, at least pick your next floor covering with care. Take the time to find one that is as chemically safe and easy to clean as possible. And if you or members of your household have an allergy to dust mites, endeavour to buy from a retailer who understands your specific needs.

Excellent carpet alternatives include polished hardwood, natural linoleum (not to be confused with vinyl), natural rubber tiles, polyolefin (a type of plastic), ceramic tiles, and stone, such as granite, sandstone, limestone, slate, quartzite and marble.

MAINTAINING AN EXISTING CARPET

◆ Vacuum frequently using a machine with an extra-thick bag and good suction – it should be powered to the tune of 1,000 watts. Fit an exhaust microfilter to your existing vacuum cleaner if it does not already have one to prevent dust from being blown back into the air. Better still, use a unit fitted with a high-efficiency particulate air filter (HEPA) or one with an electrostatic filtration system.

◆ Dry steam-cleaning reduces dust mite populations, but experts believe the results to be short-lived. Also, some treatments are not sufficiently powerful to reach mites buried deep in the pile. Remember to vacuum up the dead mites and denatured allergens after steam treatments.

◆ Do not clean your carpet with 'wet' steam or hot water. Anything that leaves carpet fibres moist provides a perfect environment for further dust mite colonisation, as well as the formation of mould and mildew. Whereas professional cleaning machines remove both dust and cat allergens, domestic models tend to blow fine water droplets containing dissolved allergen back into the air.

◆ Dispose of wet carpet. Mould contamination occurs very fast and is difficult to control, unless you resort to chemical treatments.

◆ Insist that people remove their shoes. Dust, dirt and pesticide residues can be tracked in from outdoors and sink into carpets. Also, damp soles encourage the establishment of mould and mildew.

◆ Treatment with liquid nitrogen can reduce mite numbers significantly for a short time.

◆ Seal your existing carpet with a non-toxic floor seal or a vapour barrier. These products are usually sprayed on and left to dry, forming a protective layer that stops harmful materials from outgassing.

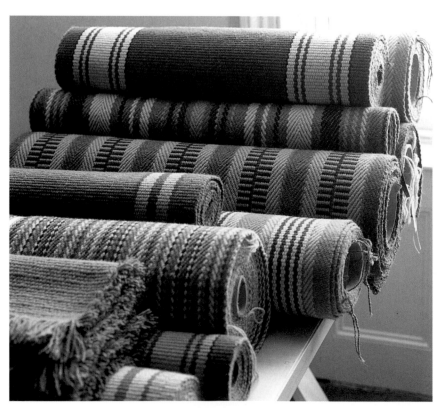

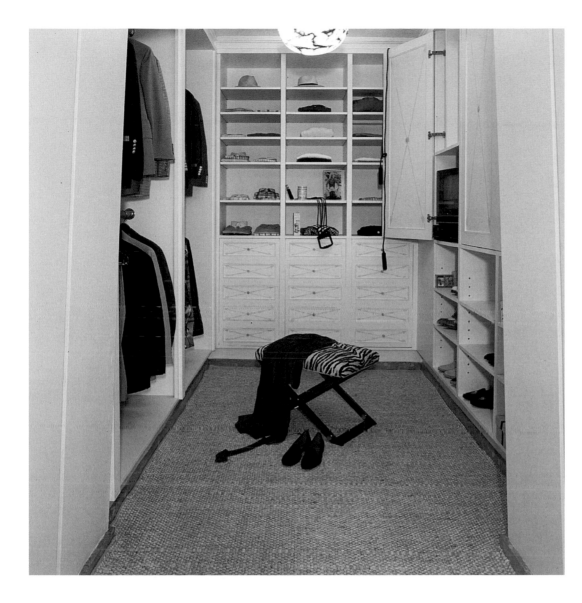

FAR LEFT For allergy-sufferers, scatter rugs are preferable to wall-to-wall carpet. Even where allergy is not an issue, rugs have the advantage of not emitting toxins from glues and underlay.

LEFT For a modern look choose natural fibres such as seagrass, sisal or coir. Dust mites hate these prickly fabrics, and their short pile makes them easier to clean thoroughly with a vacuum cleaner.

BUYING A NON-TOXIC CARPET

◆ Opt for natural fibre carpets over synthetics. Good carpet materials include cotton, seagrass, sisal, coir (coconut-husk fibre) and wool, though you may want to bear in mind that dust mites feast on wool. Try to ensure the carpet has a dense, tight weave, to inhibit the build-up of excessive dust. Also, favour wool carpets that have been woven directly onto a linen and cotton base.

◆ Choose a carpet that has not been treated with chemicals during the production process. Natural carpets are often anti-static because they contain no man-made fibres. And if the lanolin from the wool fleece is still present, this will act as a natural stain inhibitor. Untreated wool carpet is undeniably hard to find; however, some companies are putting a lot of effort into new approaches to the problem of moth attack.

◆ Insist on backing and underlay that is made from natural fibre. Choose underlay pads made from felt, natural rubber, recycled rags, hessian or wool that has not been chemically treated.

◆ Insist that carpets be secured either with staples or a solvent-free, low-VOC adhesive, such as a natural steam-treated latex glue. Tackless gripper strips can be used at room perimeters.

◆ Where possible, ask retailers to air new carpet for a few days before delivering it. The chemicals that outgas from new carpeting drop off significantly after several hours. If this is not an option, avoid a newly carpeted area for several days after the carpet has been installed and keep the room well ventilated.

◆ Before disposing of an old carpet, vacuum clean it thoroughly to avoid dust and other contaminants being released into the air while it is being pulled up. Vacuum the area underneath to get rid of accumulated dust too.

BUYING ANTI-ALLERGY CARPETING

◆ Short pile is easier to keep clean than deep pile. This is an important consideration when dust mite allergy is a problem, as mites often become established in the deeper layers of carpeting where they enjoy some protection from vacuum cleaners and chemical treatments.

◆ Scatter rugs are better than wall-to-wall carpeting, especially those that can withstand a hot wash.

◆ For a contemporary look, choose natural fibres such as seagrass, sisal and coir, which provide prickly, inhospitable environments for dust mites.

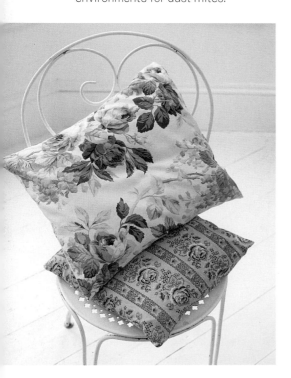

LEFT AND RIGHT Make cotton your fabric of choice for soft-furnishings. It may require more ironing than synthetic materials such as polyester, but it can be washed at high temperatures to kill dust mites and it is rarely treated with formaldehyde.

◆ Nylon carpets produce fewer airborne allergens than wool ones, possibly because the static charge generated by nylon holds the allergen particles down. So choosing a nylon carpet could mean less exposure to allergen in the atmosphere, but more exposure for babies and toddlers who are in constant close contact with the floor.

◆ There are carpets on the market that have been chemically treated with anti-dust mite agents during the manufacturing process. These agents coat the carpet fibres in such a way that the bacteria and fungi on which dust mites thrive cannot survive. However, little data is available on the toxicity of these treatments.

◆ Never attach carpet directly to concrete floors. Such floors trap moisture, allowing dust mites and mould spores to thrive.

FURNITURE, BEDDING AND CLOTHING

Many textile products are treated with formaldehyde, including all polyester/cotton-blend fabrics. The finishing process usually combines formaldehyde resin directly with the fibre, making much of it irremovable. Chemically sensitive individuals should choose natural fabrics over synthetics, both as furniture covers and as base materials for chairs and sofas, which generally contain foam. Here are some other ways to lower the chemical load:

◆ Avoid curtain and furniture fabrics that have been treated with stain-resistant coatings or flame retardants. Many companies are now starting to phase out brominated flame retardants from their products. (See also page 64.)

◆ Avoid window blinds with a PVC finish.

◆ Insist on bedding material that is 100 per cent cotton. If you are sensitive to dust mite allergens, use natural cotton sheets over allergen-barrier covers.

◆ Unless clothes are made from untreated fibres, wash them when they are new. This allows loose dye particles to be flushed away before items come into contact with sensitive skins and it reduces formaldehyde residues.

◆ Wherever possible, buy woollen garments that have not been treated with fungicides.

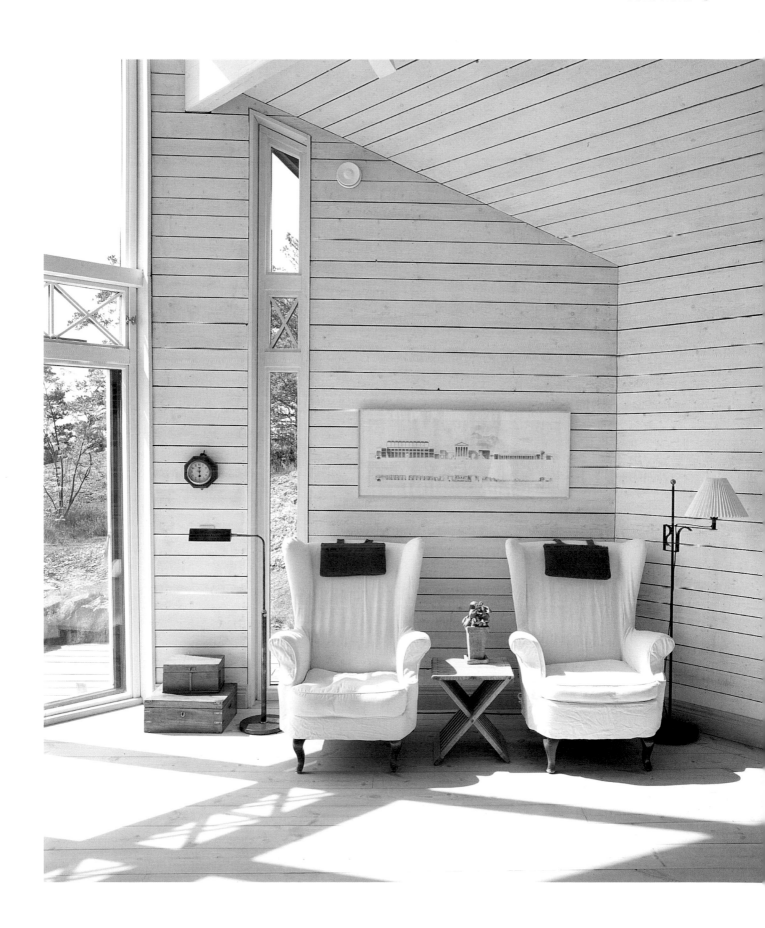

PVC (POLYVINYLCHLORIDE)

Banish PVC from your home. For virtually all PVC applications, safer alternatives exist that use traditional materials, such as paper, wood or local materials. Where these are not suitable, any other type of plastic is preferable to PVC. As a result of pressure from consumer and environmental groups, safer alternatives are already being used in the car and packaging industries and by manufacturers of building materials. Also, PVC has been withdrawn from products in the home furnishings store IKEA and was banned from facilities at the Sydney 2000 Olympic Games. In the United States, some doctors are refusing to use PVC in the context of their work, for example in surgical gloves.

WINDOW FRAMES

Avoid frames made from PVC-u, as it contains at least six highly poisonous chemicals. Instead, use less harmful polyolefin-based plastics, such as polyethylene or polypropylene. Best of all, use wood. Well-maintained, high-performance wood windows last far longer than vinyl and, over the lifetime of the windows, should not cost more than PVC-u equivalents. Buy windows manufactured with wood that comes from properly managed forests only, and take care in the choice of preservatives, paints and stains.

VINYL AND CHILDREN

Vinyl is very common in products designed for children, such as pencil cases, rain hats and coats, toys, umbrellas, backpacks, ponchos, school supplies and sports equipment. Phthalates, lead and cadmium are widely present in vinyl products, and all three can be highly dangerous. Lead is absorbed when a vinyl item is chewed or swallowed.

WALLPAPER

Vinyl wallpaper should come with the same health warnings as vinyl flooring, so avoid decorating your walls with easy-wipe vinyl paper. Also, ensure that wallpaper is applied with an adhesive that is solvent-free and, ideally, free of chemical fungicides. Ecological paste is available.

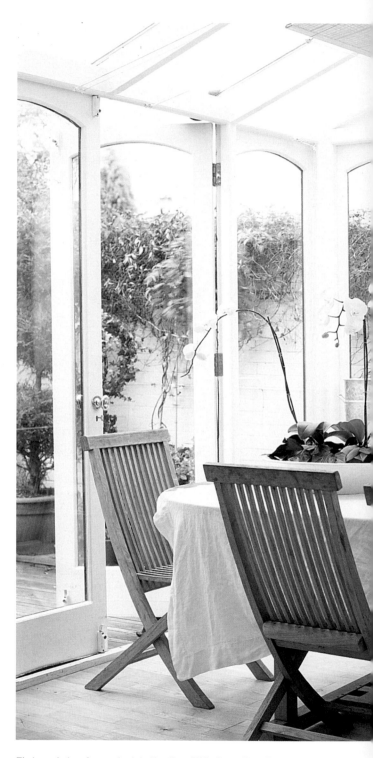

Timber window frames look better than PVC alternatives. They also last longer, and do not contain any of PVC's chemicals. But if you inherit wooden frames from a previous occupant, watch out for flaking paint; if the paint chips are old enough to contain lead, the health consequences could be serious.

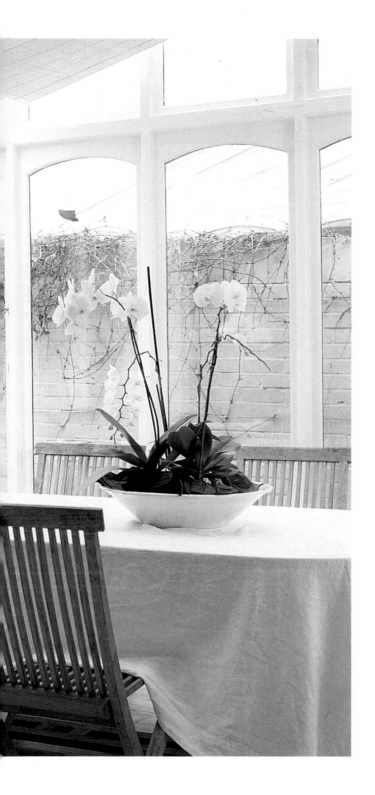

PLANTS: NATURE'S HELPING HAND

If you choose your house plants wisely and care for them properly, they will do wonders for the air in your home. Plants absorb carbon dioxide as part of their natural process of photosynthesis, and an in-depth study sponsored by NASA found that some remove airborne pollutants through both their leaves and roots. These pollutants include formaldehyde, carbon monoxide, benzene, cigarette smoke and ozone. The plants are not harmed and, providing they are looked after in the normal way, should continue to absorb chemicals for as long as they grow. Here is a list of the best potted greenery to keep in your home:

SPIDER PLANT

The common spider plant removes formaldehyde from the air. It has also been found to remove 96 per cent of carbon monoxide emissions under laboratory conditions. Keeping half a dozen spider plants in a room that has newly fitted composite-board furniture will significantly diminish the effects of formaldehyde.

MOTH ORCHID AND DWARF DATE PALM

Both remove toluene and xylene from the air. The moth orchid emits large quantities of oxygen, which stimulates concentration.

CHRYSANTHEMUM, GERBERA AND ENGLISH IVY

All three absorb benzene. Gerbera and English ivy are also effective at absorbing formaldehyde and eliminating bad smells.

PEACE LILY AND PALMS

Varieties such as yellow or areca palm (*Chrysalidocarpus lutescens*), lady palm (*Raphis excelsa*) and parlour palm (*Chamaedorea elegans*) absorb cigarette smoke.

POT CHRYSANTHEMUM, LADY PALM AND POT TULIP

These absorb ammonia-based smells from the bathroom.

FERNS

Ferns are good at absorbing moisture and are therefore suited to damp environments, such as bathrooms and kitchens. Boston fern (*Nephrolepis exaltata*) also reduces airborne microbes.

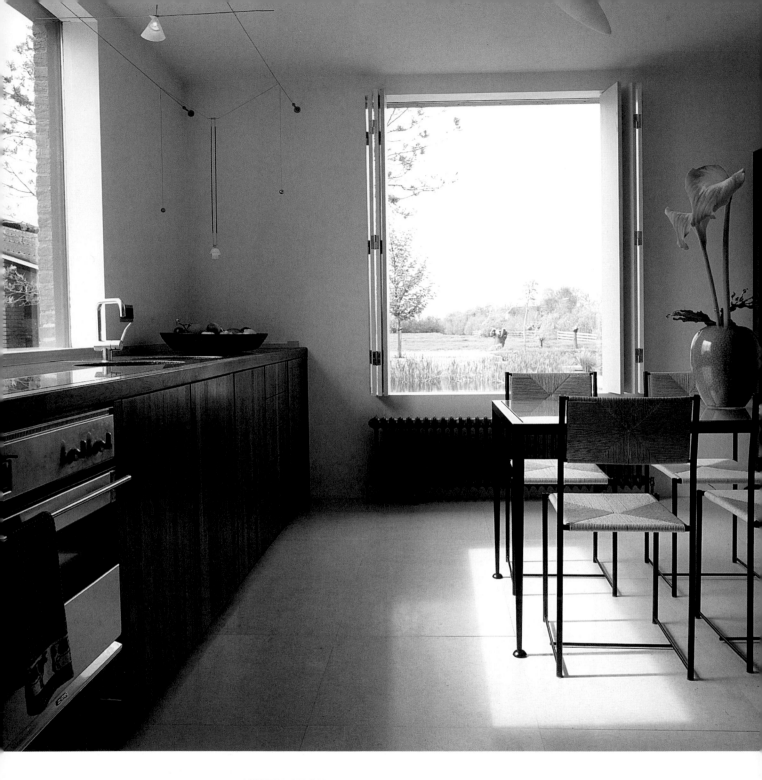

VENTILATION

One of the most effective ways to reduce indoor allergens and chemical sensitivities is to improve ventilation. The British-based Building Research Establishment recommends that houses should have a complete air change every two hours, but in today's well-sealed, energy-efficient homes, air circulates only about half as often as that.

Every room should have both rapid and background natural ventilation. Rapid ventilation occurs when a window is left open; background ventilation happens when a window is left slightly ajar, ensuring a continual supply of outside air. The same results can be achieved with a trickle ventilator: a small air grille set into the window frame.

In kitchens and bathrooms, natural ventilation may not be enough to maintain a clean, low-humidity environment, and you may need to install an extractor fan or an air filtration system.

Don't just enjoy the view from your windows: make full use of their hinges and let plenty of fresh air pour into your home.

EXTRACTOR FANS

These remove moisture as it is produced, stopping it from spreading elsewhere. Do not place an extractor fan near a window, or air coming in will go straight back out again.

SORBENTS
Air filters may contain materials called chemi-sorbents that are impregnated with chemically active materials, such as potassium permanganate or copper oxide. These react with one or more reactive gaseous pollutants, ridding them from the air.

AIR FILTERS

Air filters mechanically remove contaminants from the home; however, the evidence that modern air filters can reduce allergy symptoms is inconclusive. Some allergens, such as cat allergen, attach themselves to very small dust particles that can pass through all but the finest filters. Also, many allergens attach themselves to carpets, bedding and soft furnishings, places that are effectively out of bounds for an air filter.

Air filters come in two guises: stand-alone portable units and in-duct units installed in the central heating and/or air-conditioning system.

PORTABLE AIR FILTERS

These units are popular because they are relatively cheap and easy to move from room to room. Portable air filters range from relatively ineffective tabletop units to larger, more powerful console units. Before parting with your money, check the following:

◆ Is the unit noisy? Some portable units operating at high speed can produce noise equivalent to that made by a small vacuum cleaner.

◆ Is the unit large and cumbersome? Will it be an eyesore? And will it be easy to carry from room to room?
◆ Is the filter sufficiently powerful to service the room(s) for which it is intended?

BUILT-IN FILTERS

Filters built into your central heating system or air conditioning unit are a lot more expensive than portable units. Choose a filter according to the type of pollutant that needs to be eliminated. Filters are classified by the method employed to remove particles of various sizes from the air. Three types are on the market: mechanical filters, electronic air cleaners and ion generators. Hybrid units are also sold that use two or more of these removal methods. The following points should be considered before buying this type of filter:

◆ What are the power and access requirements of your chosen filter?
◆ What sort of maintenance does the unit require, including cleaning and replacement of filters and sorbents? (Sorbents have been developed to remove specific gaseous pollutants such as formaldehyde.)

Natural cleaning products

Two generations ago, any product formulated in a laboratory was assumed to be an improvement on what nature could offer. Thankfully, today's consumers are a lot more discerning. Nonetheless, manufacturers of household products are incredibly convincing with their claims of 'unbeatable cleaning power', and the modern home is likely to be awash with substances that have the power to undermine well-being, trigger allergic reactions and threaten future health. Most people think that they have no choice but to use powerful chemicals to keep grime at bay, but there are gentler options that do the job just as well.

One of the simplest yet most effective steps you can take in the home is to throw out all the toxic, heavy duty chemicals used to maintain it. Go back to basics with some of the cleaning products used to great effect by your grandmother.

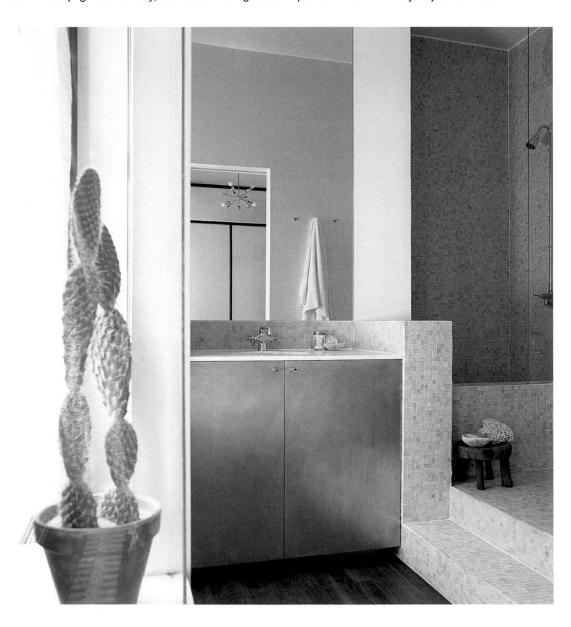

Household chemicals, it would seem, are here to stay. After all, kitchens must be cleaned, toilets disinfected, drains kept clear, dishes and clothes washed, and commercial products do these jobs nicely. But less hazardous alternatives do exist, and one of the most effective steps you can take to reduce the chemical overload in your home is to throw out all the chemicals used to maintain it.

It is encouraging to see that supermarkets are stocking a growing number of products that promise to respect both the purchaser's health and the environment. And as a rule, anything 'earth friendly' is better than a common chemical detergent. However, not all so-called ecological products are totally green; biodegradable (and therefore environmentally friendly) they may be, but only some are totally free of synthetic fragrances or petrochemical derivatives. That said, there are some excellent cleaning products on the market, though consumers must broaden their search to find them, as many are available only by mail order or in health food stores. The alternative is to create your own safe cleaning products.

HOMEMADE CLEANING PRODUCTS

There are plenty of effective cleaning formulations that can be rustled up from harmless ingredients, some of which are probably in your kitchen already. Here are some of the best cleaning ingredients to have to hand:

BAKING SODA (SODIUM BICARBONATE)

A lightly abrasive, non-corrosive material that is great for absorbing odours and for light cleaning and polishing. Available in small quantities from supermarkets and in bulk from some natural food stores.

DISTILLED WHITE VINEGAR (ACETIC ACID)

Useful for removing limescale, grease, and odours. Buy the cheapest bottle you can get hold of.

LIQUID SOAP

Castile and vegetable oil-based soaps have excellent cleaning power. Available from good health food stores and by mail order.

BORAX (SODIUM BORATE)

A naturally occurring mineral, borax is good as a stain remover for clothes and as a scrubbing compound for general cleaning purposes, but not 100 per cent safe. It is a dermal and respitory irritant and may have toxic effects on human reproduction. Available at chemists and some supermarkets.

SODIUM HEXAMETAPHOSPHATE ('GRAHAM'S SALT')

This naturally occurring mineral gives extra punch to other natural cleaning ingredients. It is non-toxic to humans, although it is corrosive to the skin and should be kept out of the reach of children. As an environmentally unfriendly phosphate, it should be used sparingly. Available by mail order.

WASHING SODA (SODIUM CARBONATE)

Sodium carbonate cleans clothes, softens water, cuts grease, and increases the cleaning power of soap. It is often available as crystals from large pharmacies and hardware stores.

CORNSTARCH

Cornstarch starches clothes and absorbs oil and grease. Available from supermarkets.

LEMON JUICE

Freshly squeezed lemon juice cuts through grease and removes perspiration and water stains from clothes.

GENERAL HOUSEHOLD AND BATHROOM CLEANING

You can do a surprising amount of housework – and certainly all of your damp-dusting and window-cleaning – with a blend of 50 per cent vinegar and 50 per cent water. If you need something a little stronger, you can't go far wrong with a pint of water to which you have added 4 tablespoons of liquid soap and 6 tablespoons of baking soda or 4 tablespoons of borax. (Test the proportions until you find the formula that works best for you.)

AIR FRESHENER

There is very little in most commercial air fresheners and room deodorisers to justify their sunny packaging. Why not take advantage instead of nature's many wholesome alternatives? Here are a few suggestions:
◆ Burn essential oils instead of using sprays or plug-in deodorisers.
◆ Sprinkle borax in the bottom of your rubbish bin to inhibit the growth of odour-producing mould and bacteria.

DRAIN CLEANERS

Many commercial products are highly toxic and should be avoided. If plunging doesn't dislodge the obstruction there are a number of common ingredients with the power to flush problems away. Here are a few suggestions, starting with the mildest:
◆ Dissolve 2 tablespoons of borax in 1 litre of hot water and pour the mixture down the sink or drain to remove grease and prevent odours.

Society has become obsessed with anti-bacterial cleaning products. The truth is that household disinfectants contain a number of dangerous volatile chemicals, including the highly toxic cresol, which can cause damage if inhaled while the product is being used.

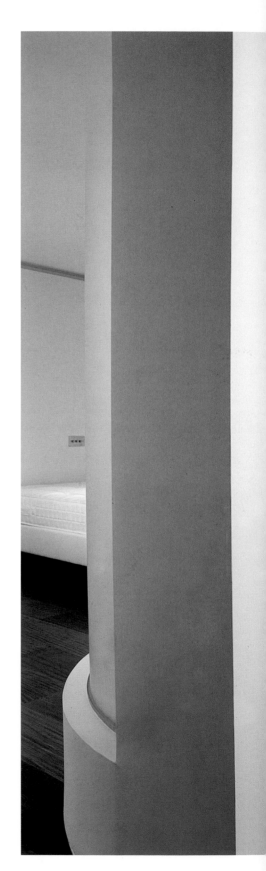

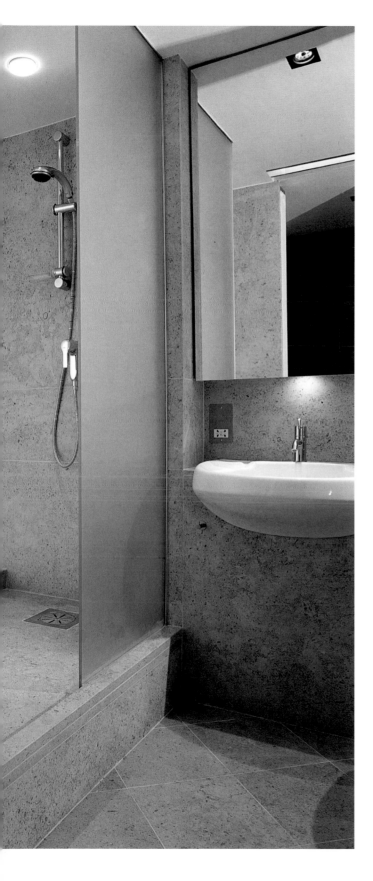

◆ Pour a handful of baking soda and about 125ml of white vinegar down the drainpipe and cover for one minute. Rinse with hot water.

◆ If all else fails, pour about 60ml of 3 per cent hydrogen peroxide down the drain, give it several minutes to react, then plunge. You may need to repeat this process.

FURNITURE AND FLOOR WAXES AND POLISHES

These may appear harmless enough and some even give off a rather pleasant aroma, but most waxes and polishes release harmful fumes. It is the additives that make polish potentially harmful, so do away with all the undesirable extras by purchasing a bottle of plain mineral oil, which is the active ingredient. Mineral oil is sold in good hardware stores. Here are some more ideas:

◆ Add a squeeze of lemon juice to a small cupful of mineral oil to give your polish a citrus zing.

◆ Oak polish: Add half a tablespoon of sugar and a table-spoon of beeswax to half a litre of beer and bring to the boil. Allow to cool, then wipe onto wood. When dry, polish with a soft cloth or chamois leather.

◆ To hide scratches on a wooden surface, rub with the flesh of a walnut.

OVEN CLEANERS

Commercial oven cleaners are extremely potent chemicals. Anyone would benefit by avoiding them, but asthmatics in particular should steer clear – reactions can be sudden and severe. A paste made from baking powder and warm water makes an excellent alternative.

MOULD AND MILDEW CLEANERS

Use a mixture of borax and water in a spray bottle. If you have a mould problem in the bathroom, try washing down the walls with a borax solution and leaving it on: borax inhibits mould growth. Also, coating the base of shower curtains with Vaseline or baby oil is another effective measure for inhibiting mould formation.

CARPET AND UPHOLSTERY SHAMPOOS

Here are some recipes for homemade cleaners that will not leave you wheezing and sneezing:

◆ Dirt stains: A borax–water solution (try 60ml borax to 750ml water) works wonders.

◆ Red wine: Blot up the worst of the liquid, rub baking soda into the stain. Leave to dry and then vacuum.

◆ Oil: Cover with cornstarch, leave overnight, then vacuum it up.

ABOVE To keep your kitchen spotlessly clean, wipe surfaces frequently with hot water and a mild soap. Microbes only proliferate when wiping is infrequent and cursory.

RIGHT Try ecological cleaning balls for a bleach-free wash.

◆ Ink: Cover with cream of tartar and add a squeeze of lemon juice. Rub into the stain, brush it off, and sponge immediately with warm water. Repeat as necessary.

◆ Grease: Cover the stain with baking soda, rubbing it lightly into the surface of the fabric. Leave for an hour, then brush off.

◆ Urine: Rinse with warm water, then apply a solution of 3 tablespoons of white vinegar and 1 teaspoon liquid soap. Leave on for 15 minutes, then rinse and rub dry. Alternatively, use a diluted borax solution.

◆ To deodorise musty rugs and carpets: Cover with baking soda and a handful of lavender flowers. Leave overnight, then vacuum. Repeat if the carpet is very smelly.

DRY CLEANING

Percholoroethylene is the chemical most commonly used by dry cleaners, but it is by no means the only toxic chemical applied to fabrics. Fortunately, percholoroethylene evaporates leaving no residue, and if clothes are properly dried, there should be no problem. However, if clothes are

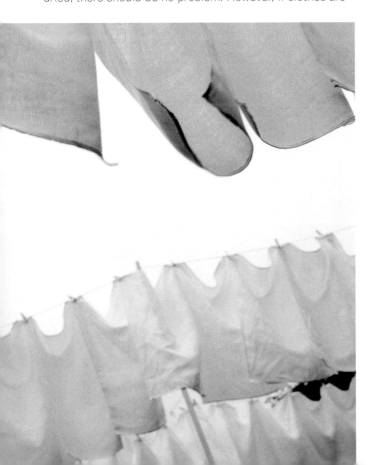

returned still damp, pollutants are released when the protective plastic is removed. (Note that clothes should always be left to dry thoroughly before being returned to the customer.) Always hang freshly dry-cleaned clothes in a well-ventilated area or a sheltered outdoor spot until the chemical smell evaporates: a couple of days should suffice. Here are two less toxic alternatives to percholoroethylene:

◆ For an all-purpose spot remover: Dissolve a pinch of borax in 500ml cold water. Sponge it onto the garment and let it dry. If the fabric can be washed, soak it in a solution of diluted baking soda, or 2 tablespoons of borax and 4 litres of water, then wash.

◆ To soften grass and milk spots, sponge glycerine onto the fabric, then rinse with warm water.

LAUNDRY DETERGENTS

Here are two excellent alternatives to the chemicals in common clothes detergents:

◆ Ecological cleaning balls: These plastic balls bounce around in the washing machine removing dirt and odours without the need for detergents or soaps. Ceramic pellets contained within each ball produce ionised oxygen that activates the water molecules, allowing them to penetrate deep into clothing fibres to lift dirt away. Each ball is reusable up to a thousand times and, because no suds are formed, consumers can save water and energy by shortening the rinse cycle. (Where there are deep stains or grease marks, borax can be added to the wash.)

◆ Replace washing machine detergents with natural liquid soap or soap flakes. To overcome the problem of soap scum, add sodium hexametaphosphate to the washload. (Halve the amount of soap used in the wash by adding sodium hexametaphosphate, available by mail order.)

DISINFECTANTS AND ANTIBACTERIALS

Piping hot water and pure liquid soap are sufficient to kill harmful bacteria in the kitchen. If in doubt, add borax or a dash of teatree oil (a natural disinfectant) to the hot water.

BLEACH AND FABRIC CONDITIONER

Before tipping a capful of chlorine bleach or fabric conditioner into your wash, try a more natural formulation.

◆ For a fragrant washload, place a handkerchief impregnated with a few drops of your favourite essential oil in the tumble drier.

◆ Chlorine bleach is the one to watch out for, so switch to the non-chlorine variety that uses sodium perborate or borax as a bleaching agent. Alternatively, use straight borax or add 2 tablespoons of sodium hexametaphosphate to the washing machine. This dissolves mineral deposits and soap scum and prevents clothes turning dull.

DISHWASHER DETERGENTS

When there is a choice, favour the ecological brands stocked by your supermarket (though some of the best green commercial products are available by mail order only). Alternatively, use sodium hexametaphosphate, which dissolves grease and leaves no water spots on glasses. If you are not in the habit of rinsing items before putting them in the machine, you will also need to add a mixture of baking soda and borax (2 tablespoons of each) to the detergent dispenser, as sodium hexametaphosphate does not dislodge caked-on food. Add about 250ml white vinegar to the rinse compartment of the dishwasher for an extra-shiny finish to your glassware.

DISHWASHING LIQUIDS

These may be marketed as harmless and even kind to your hands, but in reality dishwashing liquid is no more than liquid detergent with added dye, synthetic fragrance and perhaps a dash of ammonia. Replace your usual product with something kinder. Here are some tips:

◆ For normal dishwashing, use pure liquid soap. This will do the same job without harming you or the environment.

◆ Add a tablespoon of borax to the water, and the grease will be cut from your dishes, china and pans.

◆ In hard-water areas, add 2 teaspoons of sodium hexametaphosphate to the water and halve the amount of soap.

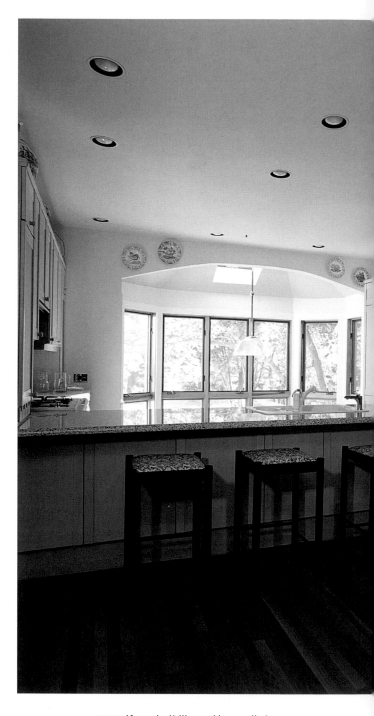

ABOVE If you don't like cooking smells to linger, there are many alternatives to air fresheners and plug-in deodorisers; burn essential oils; grow mint or basil on the kitchen windowsill; or place cloves, a cinnamon stick, orange peel or lemon rind in a pan and simmer for an hour.

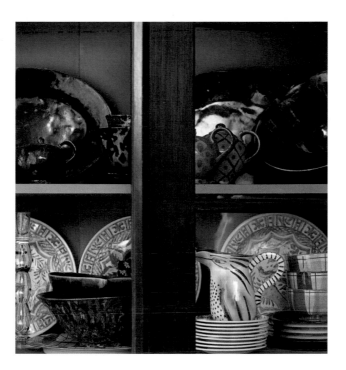

LIMESCALE

Here are two simple ways to dissolve the layers of limescale that can block shower heads. A metal shower head can be boiled for 15 minutes in a litre of water into which you have poured 125ml vinegar. To clean a plastic shower head, submerge the unit in a hot solution of 50 per cent vinegar and 50 per cent fresh water.

GLASS CLEANERS

For spotless windows and mirrors, try one of the following:
◆ Mix one part water with one part vinegar. Spray it on glass, then wipe off with a dry cloth or crumpled newspaper. This solution works well but if you end up with streaks, put it down to a build-up of wax from your regular cleaner. Remove this film by rubbing a little pure alcohol over your windows.

PORCELAIN CLEANER

Rub the surface with a cloth dipped in cream of tartar.

LIMESCALE REMOVER

Soak a paper towel in vinegar and leave it draped over the affected area for an hour, then rinse.

AEROSOLS

If you make just one health concession to your cleaning routine, let it be this: throw away all household aerosol sprays and replace them with products sold in a liquid or solid form. Aerosols are particularly harmful to asthmatics, but they are bad for everyone else, too.

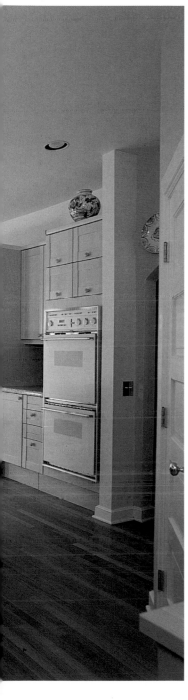

ABOVE RIGHT Keep china displays and other ornaments behind glass doors to minimise dust, and the proliferation of dust mites.

Pest control

If you simply cannot contemplate sharing your living space with things that creep, crawl and buzz around your head at night, turn to nature rather than chemistry to make your home a no-go area for common indoor pests. In the first instance make insects feel thoroughly unwelcome by removing their food source, drying up their water supply by repairing dripping taps and clogged drains and throwing out clutter among which they love to hide. Next, put on your apron, roll up your sleeves, and cook up a non-toxic pesticide.

Beware of pesticides that are marketed as 'green' or 'organic'. They might contain one ingredient that is 'natural' but this may make up only a small percentage of the product and the rest may be synthetic and potentially harmful. Scrutinise labels carefully. If you must use a commercial pesticide, choose one in liquid form: powders become easily airborne and can be absorbed into the lungs. Alternatively, try sticky flypaper (brightly coloured strips work well for many airborne insects), boric acid traps, silica gel traps, electrocuters and light traps. Sprays containing hot pepper, garlic, soap and soapy lime can be extremely effective in repelling insects. Homemade pesticides are also much safer to use around pets and children. Here are a few suggestions:

ANTS

◆ To keep ants out of the house, sprinkle powdered red chilli pepper, paprika, dried peppermint or borax where they enter.
◆ Alternatively, grow mint around the outside of the house. Ants hate the smell.
◆ Flooding with boiling water or soapy water kills ants nesting beneath outdoor surfaces, such as patios and paving stones.
◆ Do not store food in screw-top jars: ants are capable of entering along the connecting threads. Use only glass food containers with rubber seals or fit lids with plastic gaskets. Plastic containers should have tight-fitting lids.

◆ Boric acid baits will be picked up by foraging ants, partially ingested and carried back to the nest. Sprinkle a small amount of the poison on food in a container with a pierced lid to provide access.
◆ A drench of household soapy water combined with pyrethrum will kill some ants and cause the remainder to move the nest.
◆ Seal off ant no-go areas (including pot plants) with petroleum jelly or a strip of duct tape: ants will not cross a sticky barrier.
◆ Protect pet dishes by placing them in a moat of water.

COCKROACHES (SEE PAGE 48)

FLIES

◆ Make your own flypaper by boiling equal parts sugar, corn syrup and water together. Dip thick paper into the cooled solution, let any extra solution drip into the sink, then hang the paper in your chosen spot. Flies are instantly drawn to the sweet treat and are trapped.
◆ Hang cloves around the room or scratch the rind of an orange or lemon to deter flies. They cannot abide the smell.

MOSQUITOES

There are a number of herbal insect repellants on the market, many of which contain citronella oil. If you prefer to make your own, here are some simple solutions:
◆ Rub vinegar onto exposed skin.

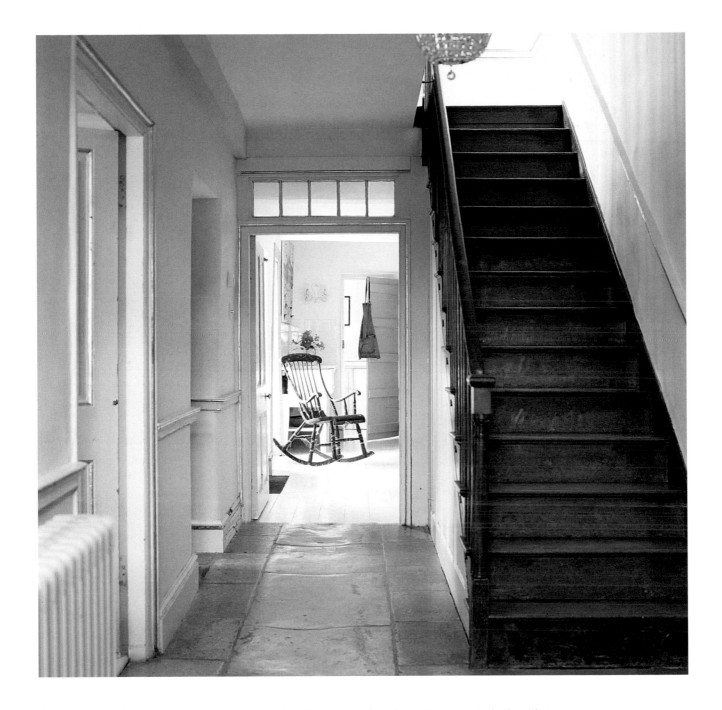

If ants doggedly colonise your home, lay traps containing boric acid (a naturally occurring mineral of lower acute toxicity than other insecticides) where they are likely to travel. This poison will be partially ingested in the ants' stomachs and then passed on to other members of the colony on return to the nest.

◆ Mix a few drops of the following essential oils with a vegetable oil base: penny royal, citronella, peppermint, eucalyptus, rosemary and tansy. Shake well and apply small amounts to the skin, as if dabbing on perfume. Avoid getting the mixture into eyes, and store away from heat.

◆ Burn citronella candles.

◆ Grow basil outside your windows. This deters mosquitoes from entering.

RIGHT When the weather turns warm, wash your winter woollens to kill any moths, then store them with a natural insect repellant in closed cupboards.

MOTHS

Thankfully, there are a number of alternatives on the market to the traditional, ultra-smelly variety of moth crystals. They are sold in large department stores and some dry cleaners, and usually contain a herb such as lavender or the oil, chips or needles of cedar. One of the best things about these natural alternatives is their scent, which is as pleasant to us as it is repellant to moths.

◆ Make moth-repellant sachets from dried lavender, or equal parts dried rosemary and mint.

◆ Wash moth larvae out of your clothes before storing them for the summer. The moths that cause damage to your clothes are too small to see, and it is actually their larvae that eat the fabric.

◆ Vacuum-pack your clothes. A number of plastic-bag systems are available that hook up with a vacuum cleaner.

HEAD LICE

These lice live exclusively on the human head, feasting on human blood. As they do not fly, they are transmitted by close head contact. The bites are not painful, but lice saliva can cause allergic reactions that result in itching. Scratching can damage skin and serve as an entry for germs. Children aged four to 16 are most likely to be

INSECT REPELLANTS

The insect repellant pyrethrin is derived from pyrethrum, an extract from the crushed dried flowers of *Chrysanthemum cinerariifolium*. The synthetic version is called pyrethroid. Though poisonous to insects and deadly to fish, both pyrethrin and pyrethroid are of low acute toxicity to mammals. The problem with shop-bought formulations is that they contain other dangerous pesticides. A safer option is to buy pyrethrin powder by mail order and to use it in its pure form.

afflicted, but lice often spread throughout a family. There is no shortage of powerful chemicals on the market designed to control lice, though there is growing concern over their toxic effects on youngsters. A non-toxic alternative is to smother the lice by rubbing olive oil into the hair, covering the head with a showercap, and leaving overnight.

ANIMAL FLEAS

The most common species is the cat flea, though the dog flea is fairly common as well. Eggs are laid on the cat or dog host and the hatching larvae drop off into rugs, blankets, furniture and between cracks in the floor. Cat fleas cannot survive on humans alone, but they bite freely. Most bites occur from mid-calf down and usually appear as small red bumps, usually with three or four in a line. Some people (and pets) have allergic responses to flea bites. When a flea problem arises, avoid toxic collars, soaps, dusts, sprays and 'bombs'. Instead, try one of the solutions suggested by the US National Coalition Against the Misuse of Pesticides:

◆ Vacuum rooms daily and change the collection bag often.

◆ If you are going away from home for two or three days, leave a lamp on the floor with the bulb facing directly into a container of soapy water. The fleas will be attracted to the light and launch themselves into a watery grave.

◆ Apply an insecticidal fatty-acid soap.

◆ Repel fleas with a shampoo or spray containing limonene, an extract from citrus fruit.

◆ Sprinkle diatomaceous earth (found in garden centres and hardware stores) sparingly onto rugs and upholstery where pets lie. This abrades the flea's outer shell causing it to dry up and die. Care should be taken not to inhale the dust.

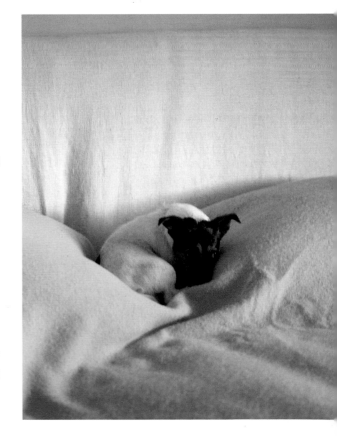

BELOW If you are in the habit of letting your pooch sleep on your bed, you may be interested to learn that dog fleas are not averse to taking a chunk out of human flesh.

Water

The quality of the water that gushes from British taps must comply with 57 parameters laid down in European law, the details of which can be found on the following website: www.dwi.detr.gov.uk. If you have a comment or query to make about the standard of water coursing through your taps, contact your local water company.

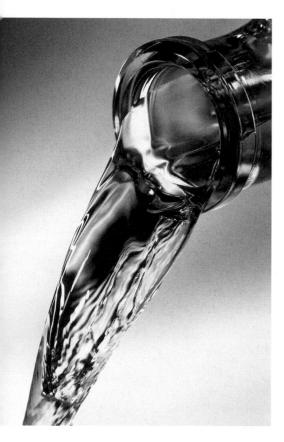

ABOVE If you suspect that your property has lead piping, drink bottled or filtered water.

RIGHT The chances are that by the time rain water flows into your kitchen sink, it will have lost much of its purity. Sediment, heavy metals, and chemicals from industry and agriculture are all picked up along the way.

Lead piping was standard until the 1970s when this dangerous metal was found to leach into the water supply. Today, nearly all the piping that links water reservoirs to the perimeter of privately owned properties is made of plastic, cement or metal. (Lead was removed from petrol and soldered cans during the same period.) However, it is the responsibility of individual home-owners to update the piping that connects the street to their residential taps. So, if your building was constructed before 1970 and no one has given the matter any thought, chances are your water is not lead-free. This being the case, you are strongly advised to employ a plumber to replace your piping (especially if you are a habitual drinker of unfiltered water).

BOTTLED WATER

Bottled water is usually sold in three types of container: glass, a type of plastic called PET (polyethylene terephthalate) and PVC (polyvinylchloride), which is often opaque. Environmental groups such as Greenpeace advise consumers to buy glass bottles as a first choice, and to avoid PVC bottles, as the risk of toxic chemicals leaching out of the plastic into the bottle is too great to ignore. Also, PVC cannot be recycled.

People opt for bottled water both because they think it tastes better than tap water and believe it to be cleaner. However, consumers are sometimes misled on this second point, as purity varies significantly from one bottle type to the next. Here is a brief lesson in label-reading to help you buy the right bottled water.

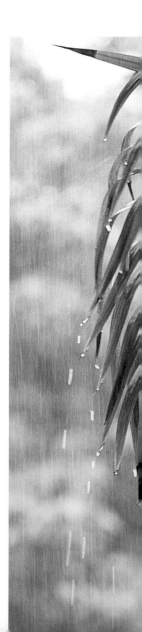

TABLE WATER

The term 'table water' describes bottled drinking water that comes from more than one source. Bottling companies are permitted to carry out processes that amend the water's constituents before the water is sold, and sometimes mineral salts are added. What a lot of consumers don't realise is that table water is often filtered tap water. This is not a bad choice if the water source is dependably clean and/or the bottlers use appropriate filters to purify it even further. However, some table water contains levels of fluoride that exceed those found in tap water several times over. Other bottled water has been found to contain more bacteria, nitrates or sodium greater than EC rules allow.

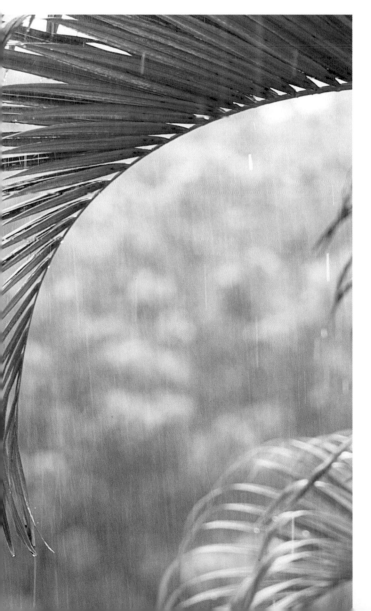

MINERAL WATER

Top of the league is natural mineral water. European law dictates that any bottle carrying this label and sold in Europe must come from a specified underground source that is protected from any type of pollution. The water must receive no treatment other than either the addition of bubbles (carbonation) or filtration to remove sand particles. It must be bottled at source and fitted with a tamper-evident seal.

SPRING WATER

Spring water is similar, except that it may receive treatment, so long as this does not interfere with its composition. Permitted treatments include filtration, ozonisation to clean it further and aeration.

WATER FILTERS

Commercial filters are not all the same. Some remove micro-organisms from the water, some remove particulates such as sand; others remove dissolved solids such as fluoride. There are essentially three types of filter on the market: distillers, reverse-osmosis devices (both of which remove particulates and dissolved solids) and activated carbon devices that remove volatile chemicals. Choose a filter according to the pollutants affecting your supply. To get your water tested, contact the Environmental Health Department who will either have their own facilities or will send you a list of analytical laboratories in your area.

Many people opt to clean their water through jug filters, which are often inexpensive and are usually capable of removing chlorine. However, they are not maintenance-free and can become contaminated if not kept scrupulously clean. A larger-scale solution to water contaminants is a point-of-device filter. Some models attach to the tap in your sink, or your shower head, and purify the water as it is used. Under-sink units do the same job, though they are out of view. There are also devices that purify water at the point where it enters your house, providing clean water from every tap.

Medicine

Mother Earth has kindly provided us with a vast palette of herbs, fruits, roots and vegetables with which to treat non-life-threatening conditions in a more gentle fashion than conventional medicine does. Here is a short guide to help you become familiar with some of the best natural health remedies. These may be particularly useful for allergy and headache sufferers who use conventional medicine on a frequent basis.

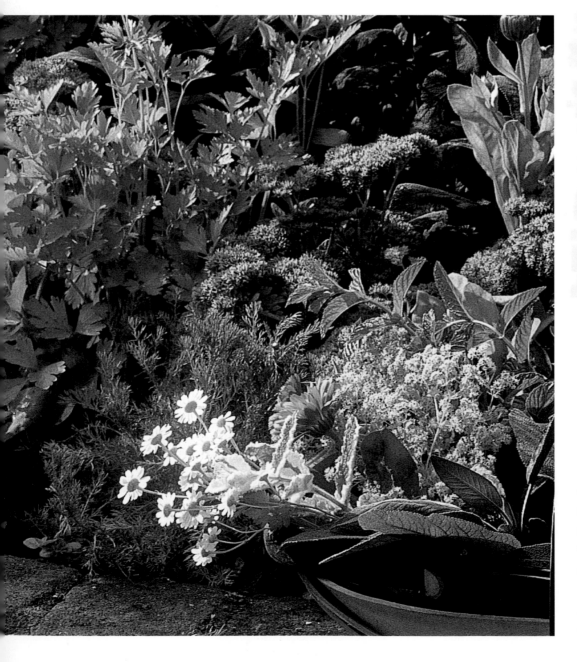

A WORD OF CAUTION
If symptoms persist or become worse, consult your doctor or allergy specialist before attempting self-medication. Pregnant women should consult a doctor before preparing remedies that involve the use of essential oils, herbs or any other natural ingredient. Some natural remedies have been linked to miscarriages.

LEFT Why pop a pill when you can take a herbal infusion to relieve your symptoms? Natural cures are often more gentle on the body and have fewer side-effects.

ABOVE RIGHT Meadowsweet is one of nature's pain-killers.

When treating a malady with natural remedies, it is vital not only to choose the best ingredients, but also to prepare them in a way that yields maximum benefits for your body. Some of the ingredients listed below are best taken in the form of a tea (in which the herbs are left to infuse in boiled water, then strained into a cup), while others are most suited for swallowing as a tablet or a syrup. Readers are advised to seek advice on the safest and most effective application for each of these ingredients: specialised books offer excellent advice, as do trained assistants in stores that sell these products.

COMMON COLDS AND COUGHS

Non-prescription cough suppressors are not intended for long-term use, and should not be used at all by people with asthma, emphysema and other lung conditions. Suppressors work by depressing the activity of the cough centre in the brain, temporarily inhibiting the impulse to cough. Other cough medications relieve irritation in the throat and bronchial passages to lessen the need to cough.

One of the best remedies for cold-related coughs is to shorten the life of the virus that brought it on. Do this by taking lots of vitamin C each day for the duration of the cold. Some people believe their colds and coughs are shortened by sweating them out with hot and spicy soups and drinks. However, if you have a persistent cough, see a doctor. Asthma may be the underlying cause of any cough that lasts several weeks, and no self-medication is appropriate.

COLDS

◆ Immune-stimulant herbs include Asian ginseng, echinacea, goldenseal, hyssop, linden and wild indigo.

◆ Natural medications with suspected antiviral qualities include zinc, elderberry, goldenseal, horseradish, myrrh, Oregon grape, usnea and wild indigo.

◆ To reduce nasal stuffiness, add a few drops of peppermint or eucalyptus oil to a hot bath.

◆ Meadowsweet is a valuable source of salycylic acid (aspirin) and relieves aches and digestive disorders.

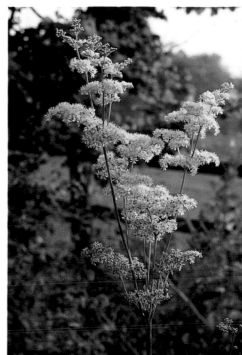

COUGHS

◆ Ingredients known to relieve bronchitis and other mild conditions include: wild cherry, marshmallow, sundew and coltsfoot.

◆ For irritating coughs try usnea or slippery elm.

◆ To treat dry, spasmodic coughs, try thyme (best combined with sundew).

CONSTIPATION

If eating prunes and other dried fruit doesn't bring relief, try psyllium husks – another natural substance that works as a safe and effective laxative. Mandrake, fenugreek, flax seeds, licorice, senna leaves, cascara bark, and aloe latex are all regarded as natural laxatives, although aloe is very potent and should be used with caution. Research suggests that chlorophyll, the substance responsible for the green colour in plants, may relieve a number of gastro-intestinal problems, including constipation.

HEARTBURN AND INDIGESTION

An effective, natural alternative to antacids is sodium algenate tablets, sold in health food stores. Wild marjoram is said to be excellent for dyspepsia, colic and wind, and to strengthen the stomach. Camomile is thought to promote normal digestion and is effective in relieving inflamed or irritated mucous membranes of the digestive tract. Peppermint, fennel seeds and roots, and caraway are also said to relieve indigestion.

INSOMNIA

The following herbs are believed to be effective promoters of sleep: lady's slipper, camomile, valerian roots, catnip, skullcap, passionflower, lemon balm, St John's wort, kava, and hops. The essential oil of lavender is calming and can also be helpful in some cases of insomnia. Many people find that drinking a tea made from lavender flowers is as effective as taking a tranquilliser. For others, a glass of milk works wonders. Milk contains the amino acid L-tryptophan, which is converted by the body into the sleep-inducing chemical messenger, serotonin.

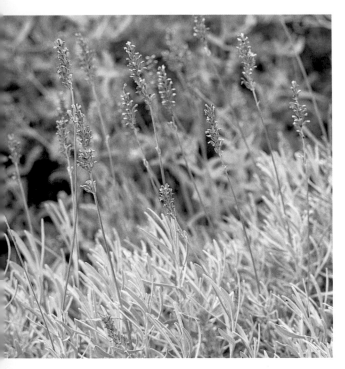

ABOVE Lavender has excellent tranquillising properties and is known to promote sleep.

ABOVE RIGHT Herbal teas can be made at the start of the day and stored in the refrigerator for a cooling drink.

NAUSEA

Catnip and sweet balm are widely regarded as excellent herbs for calming nausea. Hot peppermint or spearmint tea is said to strengthen and settle the stomach. Fennel and caraway are also known to bring relief for many people. Arguably the best natural remedy for nausea and morning sickness is root ginger.

PAINKILLERS

Painkillers are the most commonly used non-prescription drugs, but both paracetemol and aspirin can have adverse effects on some people. Aspirin is particularly potent and can interfere with blood clotting. It can also trigger or aggravate peptic ulcers as well as cause bleeding in the stomach. Both drugs are capable of triggering allergic responses.

Some herbal infusions are regarded as extremely effective at reversing or inhibiting a headache. Herbs that have proved effective when taken as a tea include catnip, peppermint, rosemary, sweet balm, blue violet, rhubarb, thyme, vervain, elder, marjoram, calamine and holy thistle. To lower a temperature, try yarrow, vervain, boneset or barberry berry tea.

ALOE VERA

The anti-inflammatory and antihistamine properties of aloe are said to be effective at alleviating the discomfort of eczema, rashes, sensitive skin, burns, acne, piles, shingles, thrush, boils, wounds and chicken pox. This natural ingredient is derived from a succulent plant, a member of the lily/onion family, and is sold both as a skin preparation and a juice. Aloe vera juice can help asthmatics and people suffering from Chronic Fatigue Syndrome.

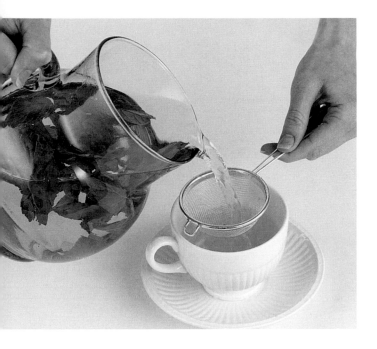

NAPPIES

If health concerns are not enough to convert you to 'green' nappies, expense could be a second motivation: washables are likely to cost less in the long run. Today, cloth nappies come in various shapes and sizes, with stretchy leg cuffs and waistbands, and press studs or velcro fastenings. Solid waste is collected in biodegradable sheets and thrown away (booster pads can be added for extra absorbency), and the cloth itself, which is usually soft and breathable, can either be cleaned and sterilised in the washing machine at home or sometimes even collected from your door by a special nappy cleaning service. (Avoid water-proof outer pants made of PVC.) If you really can't stomach converting to cloth nappies, try one of the new brands of environmentally friendly disposable nappies, free from gels, perfumes, dyes and bleaches (but a little stiff).

Cayenne pepper added to a small amount of warm water, milk or preferred tea is also said to help fight headaches. Some migraine sufferers swear by the herb feverfew; other people find relief from a sinus headache by drinking a cup of nettle tea.

ALLERGY TO DRUGS

If you suspect you are allergic to a drug, ask an allergy specialist to identify the offending substance by doing a skin prick or patch test. (See pages 36 and 37.)

◆ Once an allergy to a drug has been diagnosed, accept that you will probably never be able to take the offending substance again. However, in nearly every case an effective alternative exists.

◆ If you are allergic to aspirin, always avoid medications containing aspirin and acetylsalicylic acid.

◆ If you are allergic to any drug, consider wearing a bracelet revealing this information. This could save your life during a medical emergency.

◆ If the drug to which you are allergic is unavoidable, consider embarking on an immunotherapy programme (see page 41). This may be essential, for example, if you are diabetic and allergic to insulin.

COSMETICS AND FOOD ALLERGIES

Anaphylaxis has been reported as a result of skin contact with a food allergen, and itchy rash, urticaria, sneezing, wheezing or shortness of breath are common. Many allergenic ingredients are used in cosmetics and beauty products, but their presence is often disguised by arcane language. The International Nomenclature of Cosmetic Ingredients has standardised the names of all ingredients found in cosmetics, including food derivatives. Unfortunately, the language used in this standardisation exercise is an eighteenth-century reworking of Latin. Here are a few important components from the lists:

◆ **Egg:** *Ovum*
◆ **Milk:** *Lac*
◆ **Peanut oil:** *Arachis hypogaea*
◆ **Almond:** *Prunus amygdalus*
◆ **Walnut:** *Juglans regia/nigra*
◆ **Brazil nut:** *Bertholletia excelsa*
◆ **Hazel nut:** *Corylus rostrata/americana/avellana*
◆ **Sesame seed:** *Sesamum indicum*
◆ **Pea:** *Pisum sativum*
◆ **Coconut:** *Cocos nucifera*
◆ **Mixed fish oil:** *Piscum iecur*

BEAUTY PRODUCTS

If you have visited your local health food store recently, you may have been struck by the amount of shelf space now dedicated to hair and beauty products sold under a 'green' label. Although these products do provide a degree of naturalness, it is worth noting that few are totally natural and many contain at least some petrochemical derivatives. An alternative is to purchase natural raw ingredients and make your own beauty products.

BELOW AND RIGHT There are few substances more deeply moisturising than pure oil. All natural oils combine well with essential oils, so you can create your own personal moisturiser by adding a couple of drops of favourite oils to homemade preparations.

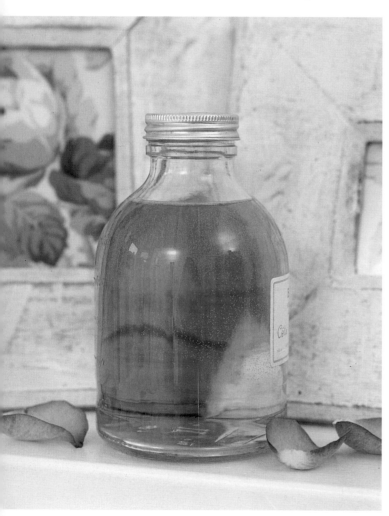

DEODORANTS

Choose deodorants that work by inhibiting the growth of odour-forming bacteria on your body, and not by covering up or clogging your pores. Avoid those that contain aluminium chlorohydrate.

ASTRINGENTS AND TONERS

Replace alcohol-based formulations with vodka, which does exactly the same job without drying the skin or causing skin reactions. Cold camomile and mint teas dabbed on the skin have the same gently astringent effect.

MOISTURISERS

Dab olive oil on your skin for a nutritious burst of moisture. If you prefer not to smell like a tossed salad, try the oils of apricot (or peach) kernel, avocado, borage, or jojoba instead.

HAIR CONDITIONERS

Beat one egg yolk until it is thick and light in colour. Drizzle in ½ teaspoon of olive oil, then slowly add about 180 ml lukewarm water. Massage this into the hair, leave for five minutes, then rinse with lukewarm water.

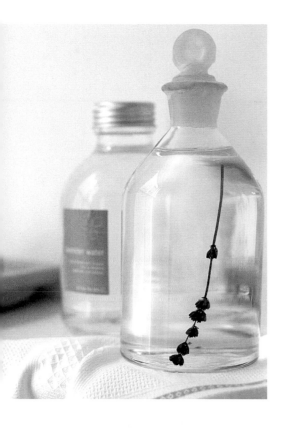

FACE AND BODY WASHES

You may know them as cleansers, complexion bars, washes, detergent or plain old soap, but there are big chemical differences among the products designed to clean your skin. Choose cleansers that contain as few synthetic substances as possible, and favour 100 per cent plant-oil soaps over all else.

Ingredients that set a good natural soap apart from its synthetic impostors include: castor oil, cocoa butter, coconut oil, natural vitamin E, tallow, olive oil and palm oil.

BUBBLE BATH

A foamy soak is one of life's little pleasures, and you can still enjoy a bubble bath without undermining your well-being. If you live in a soft water area, add a few capfuls of liquid soap close to the running water. If your water is hard, soften it by adding sodium hexametaphosphate, liquid soap, and a few drops of fragrant essential oils.

COSMETICS AND SKIN ALLERGIES

People with allergic skin conditions often turn to specialist cleaning products, creams, moisturisers and emollients to relieve some of their symptoms. Here are some tips to help anyone with eczema, chemical sensitivities or perfume allergy get the most from their merchandise:

◆ If you suffer from eczema, it would be impossible to overstate the importance of eliminating both natural and synthetic perfumes from all your beauty and cosmetic products. Not only will your condition benefit, but you will lessen your chances of developing an allergy to fragrances. (People with eczema are particularly susceptible to developing such an allergy.)

◆ Many eczema sufferers advocate the use of specialist bath oils added to warm water to soften and moisturise affected skin. It is important to pat skin dry rather than rub it with a towel. Lastly, skin must be kept moist: eczema is a dry-skin condition by definition, and it is almost impossible to massage too much emollient into affected areas.

◆ People with severe perfume allergy should avoid perfumes and perfumed products. Those with mild perfume allergy may be able to get away with using it in their hair products or on their clothes. If they suspect a product of any kind may provoke a reaction, they should test it on a small area of skin before using it extensively. (All children should avoid perfumed products.)

◆ Not everyone reacts to the same ingredients in suncare products, so it is worth trying various brands until the offending allergen or irritant is identified. For skin that is sensitive to chemicals or prone to eczema, only apply suncare products that are labelled hypoallergenic and fragrance-free. Avoid sunscreens with a high alcohol content regardless of skin type, as alcohol is highly drying to the skin. Favour physical sunblocks, such as titanium dioxide and zinc oxide, over chemical blocks. Physical blocks reflect the sun's rays rather than absorb them, and they rarely trigger skin reactions. For eczematous skin, try the sunblock lotion E45 that is specifically designed for sensitive skin.

Sources

USEFUL ORGANIZATIONS

The Anaphylaxis Campaign
2 Clockhouse Road
Farnborough
Hants GU14 7QY
Tel: 01252 542029 Fax: 01252 377140
www.anaphylaxis.org.uk

The Association for Environment Conscious Builders
Nant-y-Garreg
Saron
Llandysul
Carms SA44 5EJ
Tel: 01559 370908
Trade association for architects and builders. Information pack available.
Website: www.members.aol.com/build-green

British Allergy Foundation
Deepdene House
30 Bellegrove Road
Welling
Kent DA16 3PY
Helpline: 020-83038583
Website: www.allergyfoundation.com
Site includes a list of products that have received BAF's 'Seal of Approval' plus lots of helpful links.

British Lung Foundation
78 Hatton Gardens
London EC1N 8LD
Tel: 020 78315831 Fax: 020 78315832
Website: www.lunguk.org

Building Research Establishment
Former government organisation, now run privately, promoting healthier indoor living environments. Undertakes consultations and commissioned research on indoor air quality. Simple queries will be answered free of charge.
Tel: 01923 664200
Website: www.bre.co.uk

The Coeliac Society
PO Box 220
High Wycombe
Bucks HP11 2HY
Tel: 01494 437278 Fax: 01494 474349

Community Hygiene Concern
Manor Gardens Centre
6-9 Manor Gardens
London N7 6LA
Sells the Bug Buster Kit, a natural head lice treatment, and a demonstration video.
Helpline: 020 7686 4321
Website: www.chc.org/bugbusting.

Cosmetics Toiletries and Perfumes Association
Tel: 020 74918891
Website: www.ctpa.org.uk

Drinking Water Inspectorate
Customer complaints line: 020 79445956

Friends of the Earth
Runs a 'safer chemicals campaign' and provides information on chemicals in consumer products. Tel: 0207 490 1555
Website: www.foe.co.uk

The Government Stationery Office
Tel: 0970-6005522
To obtain a copy of the International Nomenclature of Cosmetic Ingredients (INCI) list, quote reference: OJEC L132 1/6/96.

Greenpeace
Provides information on unhealthy and environmentally damaging pollutants.
Tel: 020 78658100
Website: www.greenpeace.org (visit the 'chemical kitchen')

Latex Support Group
PO Box 27
Filey
Yorks Y014 9YH
Tel: 07071 225838 (7pm to 10pm only)

National Asthma Campaign
Providence House
Providence Place
London N1 0NT
Tel: 020 7226 2260 Fax: 020 7704 0740
Helpline: 0845 7010203
Website: www.asthma.org.uk

National Eczema Society
Hill House
Highgate Hill
London N19 5NA
Tel: 020 72813553 Fax: 020 72816395
Helpline: 0870 2413604 (1pm to 4pm, Monday to Friday) Call the Helpline to speak to an Information Officer; they do not offer a walk-in information service.
Website: www.eczema.org

Pesticide Action Network UK
Campaigns for safer use of pesticides and provides information about pesticide use and misuse. Tel: 020 72748895
Website: www.pan-uk.org.

The Women's Environmental Network
Campaigns on a variety of environmental issues, including 'healthy flooring'. Has compiled a list of suppliers of healthy and environmentally friendly flooring.
Tel: 020 74819004
Website: www.wen.org.uk

The World Wide Fund for Nature (WWF)
Panda House
Weyside Park
Godalming
Surrey GU 7 1XR
Tel: 01483 426444
Website: www.wwf-uk.org
Good for information on toxic chemicals. The WWF issues an excellent brochure on hormone-disrupting chemicals.

CONSUMER SERVICES, RETAILERS, AND MAIL-ORDER COMPANIES

Allerayde
Sells anti-mite barrier covers and other products for controlling dust-mites.
Tel: 01636 613444 Fax: 01636 611186

Auro
Sells natural paints and other finishes (oils, waxes, varnishes etc), all non-VOC.
Tel: 01799 543077
Website: www.auroorganic.co.uk

Eco-co products (AF)
Sells chemical-free laundry balls and other 'green' household cleaning products.
Tel: 020 87773121
Website: www.ecozone.co.uk

Eco Merchant Ltd
The Old Filling Station
Head Hill Road
Goodnestone
Nr Faversham
Kent ME13 9BY
Tel: 01795 530130
Website: www.ecomerchant.demon.co.uk

Green Baby
Sells natural products for babies.
Tel: 020 72269244
Website: www.greenbabyco.com

Greenlife Direct
Sells an extensive range of food supplements and some natural beauty products.
Tel: 020 72269244
Website: www.greenbabyco.com

Green People
Sells food supplements and natural and organic beauty products.
Tel: 01444 401444
Website: www.greenpeople.co.uk

The Healthy House
Sells anti-allergy products, barrier covers, carpets and non-VOC paint.
Tel: 01453 752216
Website: www.healthy-house.co.uk

Kingsmead carpets
Sells anti-allergy carpets with incorporated anti-mite agent, Dynomite.
Tel: 01290 421511
Website: www.kingsmead.carpetinfo.co.uk

Kinnereton (Confectionery)
Company producing nut-free products.
Tel: 020 74701914 Fax: 020 74875840

Lakeland Paints
Sells environmentally friendly paints.
Tel: 01539 732866
Website: www.ecopaints.com.

Medic Alert International
Tel: 020 7833 3034

Medi-Tag
Tel: 0121 2001616
Both companies sell SOS Alert bracelets for conditions such as anaphylaxis.

Natural Building Technologies Ltd
Cholsey Grange
Ibstone
High Wycombe
Bucks HP14 3XT
Tel: 01491 638911
Website: www.natural-building.co.uk

The Real Nappy Association
PO Box 3704
London SE26 4RX
Tel: 020 8299 4519
Website: www.realnappy.com

ServiceMASTER Ltd
Provides mite-killing and allergen-denaturing heat treatment for all household items.
Tel: 0116 2364646
Website: www.servicemasterclean.com.

TLC Pet Allergy Testing Ltd (TLC)
Outgang Lane
Osbaldwick
York YO19 5US
Tel: 0800 169 1958 Fax: 01904 411 444
Website: www.animal-allergy.com

Members of the public cannot order the test kit directly from the laboratory, as it is illegal for anyone other than a vet to extract blood from an animal. The vet will extract blood from the animal and return the sample to the TLC laboratory for IgG and IgE testing.

York Nutritional Laboratories
Sells human blood-testing kits by mail-order.
Tel: 01904 410410

USEFUL WEBSITES

www.absoluteallergy.com
Website linked to Living Allergy Free, the bi-monthly magazine produced for the British Allergy Foundation.

www.allallergy.net
The gateway to much of the web's information sites on allergies, asthma and intolerances.

www.Chemfinder.com
For information on many chemicals, including common synonyms and health information.

www.dwi.detr.gov.uk
Contains information on European drinking water directives.

www.ecomall.com
Extensive site selling every kind of environmentally friendly product under the sun. Also, a good source of reference material on allergies and anti-allergy products.

www.eczemavoice.com
Provides support for eczema sufferers and their families.

www.fbr.dk/chemaware
Chemical Awareness: a monthly non-Government-organisation newsletter on European chemicals policy.

www.gazoontite.com
US site packed with advice and products for allergen-free living.

www.pesticides.gov.uk
Pesticides Safety Directorate - Government website.

Index

ACKNOWLEDGEMENTS

I would like to thank Dr Jill Warner and Dr Tony Frew, lecturers in allergy at Southampton University; Muriel Simmons and Maureen Jenkins at the British Allergy Foundation; Dr Tom Woolley at the School of Architecture, Queens University of Belfast; Jeff Llewellyn at the Building Research Establishment; and Dr Andrew Jones at the School of Environmental Sciences, University of East Anglia.

The publishers would like to thank the following individuals and agencies for supplying images for this book:
Getty Images/Bruce Forster: 54-5. International Interiors/Paul Ryan: 51 (designer: Ann Robinson); 52 (designer: Gennifer Witbeck); 58 (architects: Kobe & Ou); 73 (designer: Eugenie Voorhees); 74 (designers: Haskins & Page); 76 (designer: Christian Liaigre); 77 (designers: Kastrup & Sjunnesson); 78-9 (designer: Bernard Donovan); 85 (designers: K. Foreman & K. Moskal); 86 (designer: Caroline Breet); 95 (architect: Jacob Cronstedt); 98 (designer: Paul Pasman); 100 (designer: Michael Seibert). José King: 6 (Art Architects & Designers); 13 (Noble Architects); 14, 15, 68-9 (Noble Architects); 70 (Rupert Carruthers Architect); 72, 88-9, 102-3 (Noble Architects). Dennis Krukowski: 45 (designer: Paul Silverman); 47 (as published in *The Farmhouse* by Bantam); 75 (designer: Mazurca); 93 (George Constant Inc.); 106-7 (Rolf Seckinger Inc.); 110 (Kate Altman Inc.). Narratives/ Jan Baldwin 8-9, 10, 12, 42, 46-7, 71, 80, 82-3, 84, 87, 90, 92, 96-7, 104, 107, 109, 111, 112-13; Narratives/Polly Wreford 64, 81, 119. Bill Sykes: 62-3, 105. Sam Tanner 53. Science Photo Library/K.H. Kjeldsen: 44-5; Science Photo Library/Tek Image: 16, 112. All other images © Breslich & Foss.

Project manager: Janet Ravenscroft
Illustrator: Trina Dalziel
Designer: Jane Forster

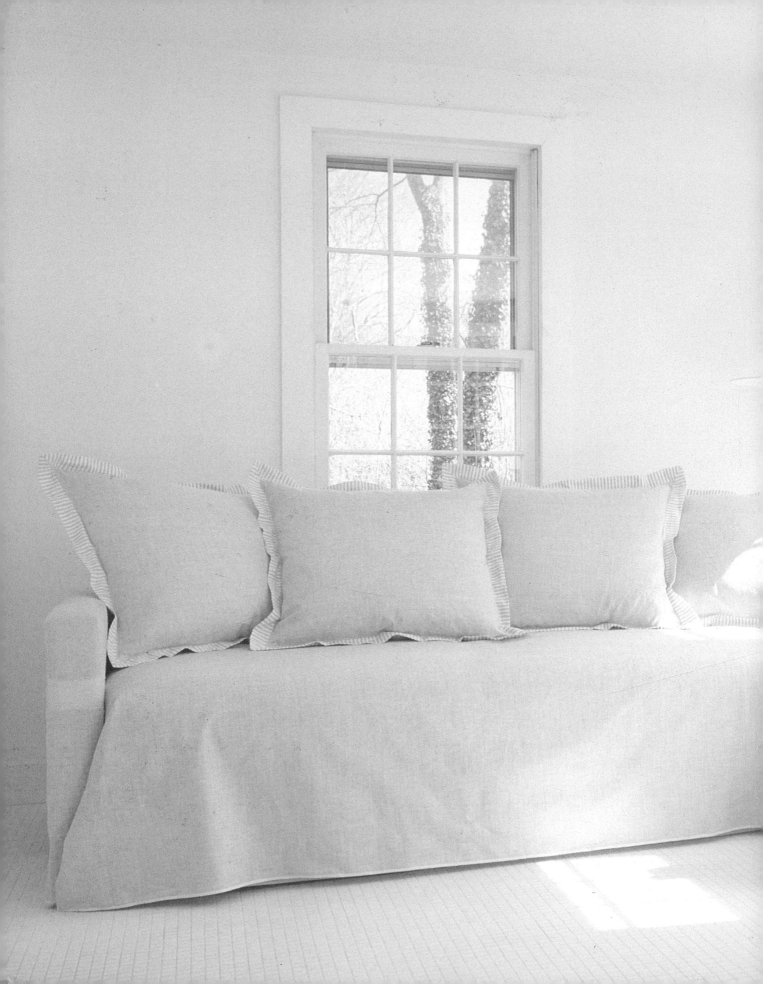